PTSponsor.com Editors

The Ultimate Guide for Foreign-Trained Physical Therapists Wishing to Work in the U.S.

Dedicated to the foreign trained physical therapists especially from the Philippines, India, Egypt and Pakistan

Rehabsurge, Inc.

The Ultimate Guide for
Foreign-Trained Physical Therapists to Work in the U.S.

ISBN: 1453854142
EAN-13: 9781453854143

Printed in the United States of America

Disclaimer:

This book is intended for informational and educational purposes only. It is not meant to provide any medical advice. Many of the product names referred to herein are trademarks or registered trademarks of their respective owners. PTSponsor.com does not warrant the accuracy or validity of the information and hereby disclaims any liability to any person for any loss or damage caused by errors or omissions in the site. PTSponsor.com also is not responsible for any material or information contained in the linked sites provided. The information presented at this site should not be construed to be formal legal advice or the formation of any relationship.

For permissions and additional information contact us:

Rehabsurge, Inc.
PO Box 287
Baldwin, NY 11510.

Phone: +1 (516) 515-1267
Email: ceu@rehabsurge.com

Rehabsurge, Inc.

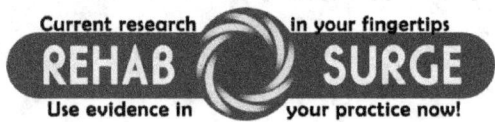

The Ultimate Guide to Foreign-Trained Physical Therapists Wishing to Work in the US

About PTSponsor.com

Founded in 2007, PTSponsor was created to provide the most up-to-date information about the Physical Therapy Licensure Process, the National Physical Therapy Exam and the Immigration of Physical Therapists into the U.S. We are dedicated to physical therapists only.

Physical therapists can easily access jobs and information all in one place. Our NPTE section provides the latest tips and reviewers available in the market. Our Immigration section differentiates between tourist visa, H1b (non-immigrant working) visa and immigrant (green card) visa. We constantly update our site for the current visa status, processing dates and case status.

Our resources section has 2 very important parts worth mentioning—best states and expense tracker. The "best states" compares the cost of living, salary and license requirements of each state. The expense tracker provides you an estimate of how much you might spend. The tracker calculates the license fees, FSBPT exam fees, English proficiency exam fees and credentialing fees.

We constantly update our articles to provide you the most recent information on –resume writing, retrogression, CLEP (College Level Examination Program), DMP (Deficiency Make-up Program), Median annual wage (salary) for all the states and much more…

Tired of spending countless hours scanning through forums to find the information you need? Visit PTSponsor.com now!

Rehabsurge, Inc.

Table of contents/Course Outline

Introduction

The Ultimate Guide to Foreign-Trained Physical Therapists Wishing to Work in the US

According to Barbara C. White (Editor: Journal of APTA), physical therapy is a health care profession that focuses on providing treatment to develop, maintain and restore maximum bodily performance. Physical therapists assess a patient's physical condition before proceeding to any treatment. Physical therapy is useful for circumstances where one's bodily performance is hindered by senility, physical injury, ailments or stress (The Encyclopedia Americana, 2003).

Physical therapists promote the quality of life by preventing injuries, deterioration, providing treatment or intervention of some motor disorders. They also rehabilitate an individual's physical performance. Treatment plans are based on a patient's medical history. A physical examination is done in order to diagnose a patient's problem (Wikipedia, 2010).

The physical therapy profession is not very popular in some countries, especially the developing ones. Those who obtained a degree in physical therapy could have limited opportunities in their own country to practice their profession. They may choose to work in more developed countries.

In the United States, there is a national shortage of Physical Therapists. The U.S. Department of Labor has designated physical therapy as a Schedule A profession. Those who are willing to work as physical therapists in the U.S. do not need to get a labor certification from the U.S. Department of Labor.

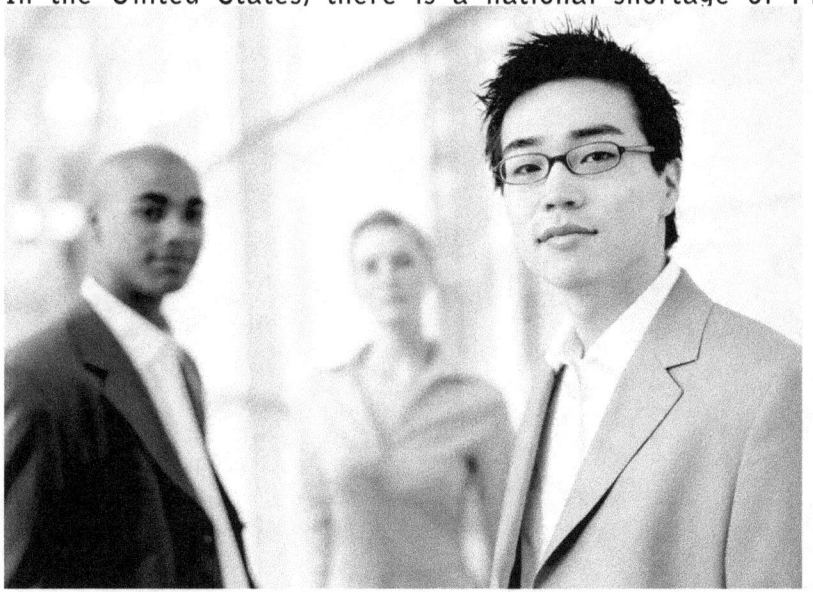

This is a very good opportunity for foreign-educated physical therapists wanting to practice in the United States, however, working overseas is a very complicated thing. A foreign-trained physical therapist should meet the educational requirements, pass the licensure examinations and visa screening. It could be very difficult for someone who has no kinship or any acquaintance in the USA.

The good news is physical therapists can find all the help they need with regards to being a physical therapist in the U.S. through this book and through PTSponsor.com. These are created to provide the latest information about the physical therapist profession. Latest updates about the Physical Therapy Licensure Process, the National Physical Therapy Examinations and Immigration of Physical Therapists into the United States can be found here.

Physical therapists can find jobs and related information in this website. The features of the site also include an expense tracker, which gives an estimate of how much is going to be spent in applying in a certain state. The "Best States" section compares the state's cost of living, salary and license requirements.

You can also take a look at the reviews. There are reviews for agencies, lawyers, states and other websites. These reviews can help you choose the best agency or lawyer.

We wish you the best!

The Physical Therapist Education

Physical Therapy education varies from country to country, or school to school. Getting a baccalaureate degree for physical therapy take four or five years. Post graduate degrees like master's or doctoral degrees may take an extra one or three years to finish. The curriculum for physical therapy consists mostly of the study of the human body, and diseases/disorders/conditions afflicting it, and its management. They are also trained to be autonomous practitioners. Through professional education, they are trained with collaborating with other health care professions (Wikipedia, 2010).

SPECIALIZATIONS

The American Board of Physical Therapy Specialties has enlisted seven certifications for physical therapists. Sports physical therapy and clinical electrophysiology is included in this list. In general, there are six typical areas of specialty with regards to physical therapy.

• Geriatric

This deals with the aging process. This is more on alleviating pains and injuries associated with aging. This type of physical therapy also aims to help older people restore their mobility and maintain their maximum fitness. Examples of diseases/conditions alleviated by geriatric physical therapy:

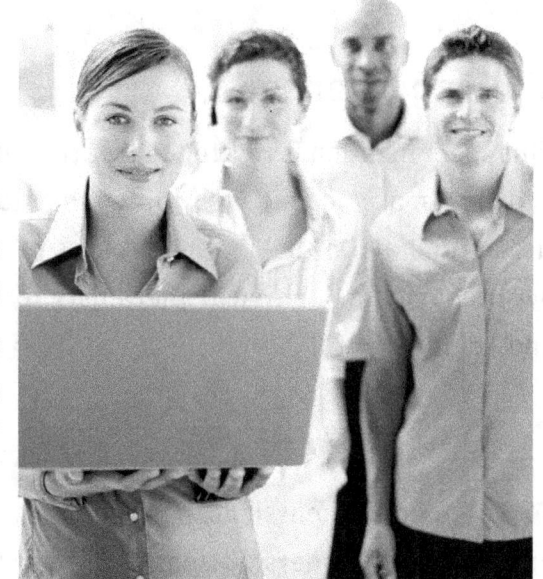

Arthritis
Osteoporosis
Alzheimer's Disease

Incontinence
Impaired Balance/Mobility

• Pediatric

Physical therapy for infants, toddlers and children involve the diagnosis and treatment of congenital or acquired diseases. Pediatric physical therapists also help in the detection and intervention of young people's health problems. Motor and cognitive skills are also improved through pediatric physical therapy. Some diseases/disorders/conditions that pediatric physical therapists manage are:

Polio
Cerebral Palsy
Spina Bifida
Torticollis
Autism
Mental Retardation
Duchenne Muscular Dystrophy
Scoliosis

• Integumentary

This specialization is related to treating the skin and other related organs. Usually, wounds and burns are managed by integumentary physical therapists. They manage necrotic tissues and aid in the healing process of wounds. Some other interventions are also used by integumentary physical therapists to improve a patient's condition, such as exercise and edema control.

• Neurological

This is a field of physical therapy which deals with individuals manifesting neurological diseases or disorders. Diseases or disorders that affect the brain or spinal cord are tackled by the neurological physical therapist. People with vision, balance, and movement impairments are also covered by neurological physical therapists, to improve or restore the patient's functional independence.

Diseases/conditions that affect the peripheral and autonomous nervous system include:

ALS
Alzheimer's disease
Parkinson's disease
Multiple Sclerosis
Brain & Spinal Cord Injuries
Stroke
Sciatica
Neuropathy
Impingement
Fibromyalgia
Radiculopathy

• Cardiopulmonary

Physical therapists specializing in cardiopulmonary PT treat individuals with cardiopulmonary disorders (such as coronary heart disease) or those who have recently undergone a cardiac or pulmonary surgery. Cardiopulmonary physical therapists aim to increase their patients' endurance and their functional independence. People afflicted with the following diseases or conditions can be helped by cardiopulmonary physical therapists.
Asthma
Coronary Artery Disease
Heart Attack
Pulmonary Fibrosis
Tuberculosis
Chronic Obstructive Pulmonary Diseases
Pneumonia

• Orthopedic

Orthopedic physical therapy focuses on the management and treatment of disorders or injuries that affects the musculoskeletal system. It also includes therapy and rehabilitation for people who had an orthopedic surgery. This type of specialization is recommended for outpatient clinics. Training for orthopedic PTs also include the treatment or management of sports related injuries, fractures, arthritis, ligament/tendon injuries. They are also trained to restore joint and spine mobility. Some examples of conditions/diseases that orthopedic physical therapists help relieve are:

Carpal Tunnel Syndrome
Tarsal Tunnel Syndrome
Rotator Cuff Tear
Adhesive Capsulitis
Piriformis Syndrome
Cervical Spondylosis

The National Physical Therapy Examination

The **National Physical Therapy Examination (NPTE)** is developed, maintained and governed by the Federation of State Boards of Physical Therapy (FSBPT), both for physical therapists and physical therapy assistants. The National Physical Therapy Examination program has three main goals:

• Give out examination services to regulatory authorities who are responsible for the regulation of physical therapists and physical therapist assistants.

• Provide a common factor in the assessment of candidates in order to compare benchmarks from jurisdiction to jurisdiction.

• Protect the interest of the public by recognizing persons who have adequate knowledge and skills in physical therapy and providing them with a license to practice their profession (NPTE Candidate Handbook, 2010).

The examination is devised to evaluate basic entry level competence of an individual who has a degree in Physical Therapy, whether it is from an accredited program or a non-accredited program equivalent to it. This examination is just a part of the evaluation process. Licensing authorities may use other supplemental assessments of the candidate's ability to practice physical therapy.

Physical therapists and physical therapist assistants belonging to the FSBPT committee are the ones who develop PT and PTA Licensure examinations. This means that a wide range of physical therapists, physical therapist assistants from different fields of physical therapy are involved in the development of the examinations. This is to ensure that the examinations are appropriate to the current practice of physical therapy.

Licensing authorities have their own criteria to give someone eligibility to take the PT and PTA examinations. A candidate must review the materials provided by the licensing authority where he/she wants to apply for licensure or certification. This is to make sure that the candidate has met the authority's requirements for eligibility.

A recent exam can be used for initial licensure, renewal/reactivation of license, or for an individual who is considered as a legitimate candidate who is not yet licensed in a jurisdiction and does not have a qualifying exam score for that jurisdiction.

Prometric administers the computer-based PT and PTA exams. FSBPT sends that score to the licensing authority. The licensing authority decides on licensure and certification procedures for its areas of responsibility. The common thing on U.S. licensing authorities is that they all have adopted the FSBPT's criteria for passing scores. This makes the minimum passing score uniform in all jurisdictions (NPTE Candidate Handbook, 2010).

The Application Process

How can you take the National Physical Therapy Examination?

1.   Request registration materials needed for taking the NPTE from the licensing authority where you choose to get a license.

2.   Complete the registration materials, and then return to the organization identified by the licensing authority. Fees will also be collected. (In completing the registration form, you will be asked to provide a Social Security Number. See Social Security Number on Chapter 4: Immigration or Chapter 2: Alternate Identification Number for more information.)

3.   The licensing authority of the jurisdiction where you wish to apply will verify and approve your eligibility. They will also notify Federation of State Boards of Physical Therapy about your eligibility.

4.   From the Federation of State Boards of Physical Therapy, you will receive an "Authorization to Test" letter. This letter contains instructions on the procedures of scheduling an appointment with Prometric. If you have any other questions about the registration process, you may email examregistration@fsbpt.org for assistance.

5.   You can now schedule an appointment with Prometric to take the NPTE. This can be done by calling the number provided from the "Authorization to Test" paperwork that

FSBPT sent you. You can also schedule an appointment online by visiting www.prometric. com. You should provide the following information to Prometric:

- Name of Examination to be taken (PT, PTA or Jurisprudence)

- Location of where you want to take the test

- Name

- Social Security Number/Alternate Identification Number

- Contact details (telephone number)

- Mode of Payment (credit card or direct debit)

6. Take the test in any Prometric testing center. You may take the test even if that is not the jurisdiction you wish to practice in. The examination has a 60-day eligibility period. That means you have to take the test within 60 days. If you fail to take the test or you have withdrawn your registration, it will lead to your removal from the eligibility list and you have to repeat the registration process again.

Preparation to Take the NPTE

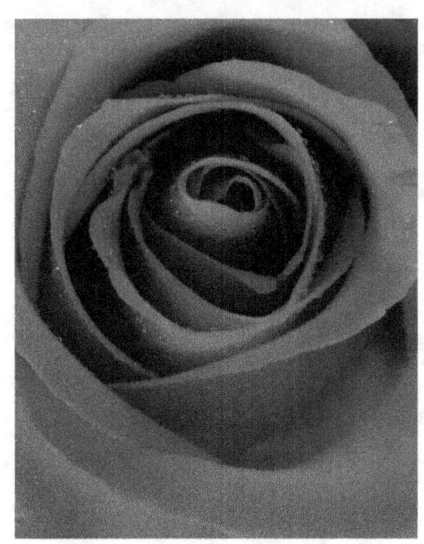

Getting a US Visa

A visa can have ambiguous meanings; it could either refer to a green card or a simple authorization to enter a foreign country. Before you can enter a country, you need to present a visa (usually a stamp on your passport) to the immigration officials.

Since the National Physical Therapist Examination is administered only in the U.S., foreign physical therapists who want to take it must get a visa first before he or she can take it. A consular officer assesses every visa application on its own merits, according to visa laws and procedures.

To apply for a visa, the steps are as follows:

1.   Complete the required application forms. Don't forget to sign it.

2.   Provide evidence that the visit to the US is only for a certain period of time and you have no intention to stay there permanently. Also bring proof that you will leave the U.S. after your legally authorized stay.

3.   Submit yourself to security clearance procedures.

THINGS TO PREPARE

1.   Application form DS-156, completed and signed

2.   Current, valid passport/travel documents

3.   Photograph (the size that is required, and the latest)

4.   Application fees and issuance fee

5.   Proof of financial capability that will cover expenses in the U.S.

6.   Proof of social and economic ties abroad

7.   Supplemental visa application form DS-157 (for men ages ranging from 16-45)

Tourist Visa for Physical Therapists

Before any entry to the United States, a citizen of a foreign country must have a Visa. Whether it is a nonimmigrant visa (for temporary stay) or an immigrant visa (for permanent residence), an alien must obtain it for security and identification reasons. There are many types of visa, the visitor visa is a nonimmigrant visa for persons who will be entering the United States temporarily either for business (B-1) or entertainment/medical purposes (B-2). For other purposes such as scholastic or journalistic, an appropriate visa must be applied since these fall under a different category. Some travelers from eligible countries may go to the US without a visa through the Visa Waiver Program.

Qualifications for a Visa

In order to obtain a visa, an applicant must pass some requirements and show that they qualify under the provisions of the Immigration and Nationality Act. The law presumes

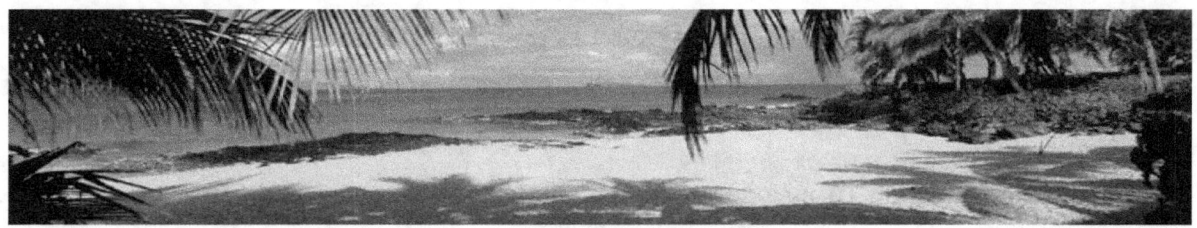

every visitor is an intending immigrant. By demonstrating the following, applicants can prove that this presumption does not pertain to them.

• The trip to the US is only for business, entertainment or medical purpose.

• Non immigrants are only staying in the US for a certain, limited period of time.

• Applicants should have a permanent residence in their country of origin, or any place outside the U.S., or have binding ties that will assure the applicant will not stay in the U.S. permanently and will go back to his or her country of origin.

U.S. Port of Entry

Applicants however should be knowledgeable that having a visa will not ensure entry to the United States. Immigration authorities have the power to deny admission, or set a time period in which a bearer of a visitor visa can stay in the U.S. Upon arrival at the port of entry, an immigration official will stamp Form I-94, Record of Arrival-Departure (notes the length of stay permitted). If a visitor wants to prolong his or her stay, beyond the time period that is stated on the Form I-94, he or she must contact the USCIS immediately to request an Application to Extend Status. This is also called the Form I-539. Only the USCIS have the authority to approve or deny the request for the extension.

10 Things you should know about the National Physical Therapy Examinations

1. Prepare two valid IDs (with pictures) such as passport or driver's license. Early arrival to scheduled appointment is recommended. Your Social Security card is not accepted as a proof of identity.

2. Examinees are going to be photographed. Thumb prints are also going to be taken. There will be a video recording of the testing sessions. The examination is computerized.

3. You are given five hours to take the examination. The examination consists of 250 items. There will be a 15-minute break, a pre-exam tutorial and post exam survey.

4. There are fifty (50) pre test questions included. Although the examination consists of 250 items, scores will be based on the 200 scored items.

5. The distribution of pre test items is random and unidentifiable.

6. Incorrect answers are not penalized.

7. The 15 minute break is scheduled after the completion of section two. The PT exam also has 3 unscheduled breaks, however, during these breaks, the timer still continues running.

8. You can mark questions you want to review before finishing a section because the testing software allows it.

9. While you are still answering a section, you can skim back and forth through it to review your marked and unmarked questions. Once you leave a section, you can't go back to review it.

10. The minimum passing score for the NPTE is 600, meaning the range is from 200-800.

Scores above 600 are considered to be passing, while those below 600 are considered to be failing by all licensing authorities.

Do's and Don'ts in Taking NPTE

Before

•	Review the materials provided by the licensing authority where you want to apply for licensure or certification.

•	Prepare documents that you will need in taking the examination as early as you can.

•	Review the course outline contained in the NPTE Candidate Handbook to be aware of the coverage of the examination.

•	Don't ask for hints from people who had taken the NPTE. Sharing recalled questions from the NPTE is ILLEGAL.

•	Arrive at the testing center as early as possible.

•	Deposit electronic gadgets (such as cellphones, pagers, digital watches, etc.) to the administering officer. Lockers are provided for examinee's personal items.

•	Don't skip your meal before taking the examination. It is not allowed to bring any food and beverage in the testing center.

During

•	Don't ask for assistance in answering the test questions.

•	If you encounter any problems with the computer you are using, notify authorized persons (the staff of Prometric). Don't try to fix things yourself.

•	Don't receive assistance from co-examinees. Once caught cheating (the whole examination session is videotaped), you will be requested to stop taking the test and leave the testing room at once. Your score will not be counted.

After

•   Don't share recalled questions to other people, whether they will take the NPTE or not. Once verified that you did so, you will ruin your chances of getting a license from any jurisdiction. Sharing test questions from the NPTE to other persons, licensing authorities, or review centers is punishable by law.

For more details, you can download the Candidate Handbook from FSBPT's website.

NPTE-i

The Federation of State Boards of Physical Therapy suspended the National Physical Therapy Examination for the year 2010 on the month of July due to a controversial leak on the examination. The said leakage on the examination was pointed to have originated

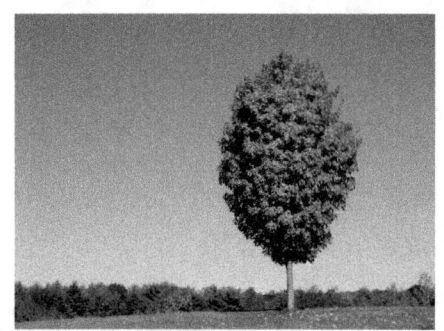

from review centers which shared recalled questions to their clients. Affected countries were Egypt, India, Pakistan and the Philippines.

The security breach was discovered and proven by forensic analysts from data regarding the performance of examinees from certain review centers. "Stark anomalies" were discovered on the test results of these candidates from some certain third-party examination security firm, and the conclusion of cheating led to the suspension of the NPTE for the mean time.

Due to this problem, the FSBPT has decided to give a new set of examination for applicants from those countries, called the NPTE-i. The NPTE-i will be given beginning 2011 twice a year to candidates from the restricted group from those countries. The FSBPT took these security measures to ensure the validity and the reliability of the NPTE. This is also to protect the interest of the public and other NPTE candidates as well. Instead of continuing the regular NPTE for these countries, FSBPT decided to develop NPTE-i which will be administered twice a year. Those who do not belong to the restricted groups (as defined by the FSBPT) are somehow affected. The registration process had a change in the availability of the Authorization to Test (ATT) letters. But they are still qualified to take the test.

Authorizations have been made available on a daily basis prior to the security breach with regards to the NPTE. Now, new authorizations will be only available once a week, during Mondays (9:00 am ET). To check your status, go to https://pt.fsbpt.net and click "Check the Status of My Request."

There is no exception to any candidate belonging to the restricted group defined by the FSBPT. Any appeals would not be heard. Candidates are advised to complete all needed documents, especially the Educational Credentials Evaluation. If a candidate is in the process of submitting requirements to his or her prospective jurisdiction, he or she must proceed so that if the NPTE-i registration opens, problems will be avoided. It must be noted that the NPTE-i will only be given twice a year and it can cause a delay if all the needed documents are not completed on time (FSBPT Suspends NPTE Examination for All Graduates of Certain Overseas Programs in Response to Pervasive Security Breaches, 2010).

TOEFL
TEST OF ENGLISH AS FOREIGN LANGUAGE

In order to work in a foreign country, you have to adjust to its language. It will be hard for you to communicate with others in that country, if you don't know their language. The Test of English as a Foreign Language (TOEFL) is given to nonnative English speakers to assess the ability of an individual's command of the English language. It is a registered trademark of the Educational Testing Service, and has a worldwide scope.

Some states may require passing the TOEFL before a foreign trained physical therapist can get a license. For green card purposes, TOEFL is also a requirement for a visa screen. If the state wherein you want to work requires passing a language proficiency test like TOEFL, then you must be ready for it.

States That Require TOEFL

Alabama	Kansas	Montana	Puerto Rico
Alaska	Kentucky	Nebraska	South Carolina
Arkansas	Louisiana	Nevada	South Dakota
California	Maine	New Hampshire	Tennessee
District of Columbia	Maryland	New Jersey	Texas
Florida	Massachusetts	North Carolina	Virginia
Georgia	North Dakota	Michigan	Washington
Hawaii	Minnesota	Ohio	West Virginia
Illinois	Mississippi	Oklahoma	Wisconsin
Iowa	Missouri	Oregon	Wyoming

Language Proficiency Examination Fees

Test of English as Foreign Language	$ 140 - $ 200
Test of Written English	$ 50 for rescore
Test of Spoken English	$ 125

TEST FORMATS

The Internet-based Test

This is a four hour test consisting of four parts. Each part measures fundamental language skills. These fundamental language skills are reading, writing, listening and speaking (About the TOEFL iBT™ Test, 2010).

- ## READING

    Description: 3-5 passages from academic texts

    Approximately 700 words long

    12-14 questions per passage

Testing Time: 60-100 minutes

Total Questions: 36-70

Score Scale: 0-30

This section of TOEFL iBT challenges one's ability to understand cause and effect relationships, comparison and contrasting and argumentation. Takers of the test should provide answers about the summary and important points from the passage. You do not have to worry if the topic of the passage is not familiar to you. The section measures reading comprehension and you don't need to be knowledgeable about the topic of the passage to answer correctly.

• LISTENING

Description: 4-6 lectures, some with classroom discussion

3-5 minutes long (each lecture), 6 questions

2-3 conversations

3 minutes length for each conversation consisting of 5 questions

Testing Time: 60-90 minutes

Total Questions: 34-51

Score Scale: 0-30

The listening section measures understanding main ideas, details, implications and cause-effect relationships. The conversations are only heard once. You can take down notes to help you in answering the questions. (You will be provided with a scratch paper). Again, some topics may not be familiar to you but you can manage if you analyze them carefully and take down the necessary details.

• SPEAKING

Description: 2 independent tasks (expressing opinion on a familiar topic); 4 integrated tasks (consist of 2 tasks involving conveying ideas from something that was read, and 2 from something that was heard)

Testing Time: 20 minutes

Total Tasks: 6 tasks

Score Scale: 0-4 points converted to 0-30 score scale

Speaking tasks evaluates an individual's skill in speaking and expressing themselves in English. It also assesses one's capability to combine and convey information efficiently using English as a language in oral communication.

• WRITING

Description: 1 integrated task (write based on something that was read); 1 independent task (support an opinion on a topic)

Testing Time: 60-100 minutes

Total Questions: 36-70

Score Scale: 0-30

The integrated task requires summarizing the topic and explaining the relation of key points. The independent task requires the examinee to write an essay that contains his or her stand on an issue, and explain why it is so. The answer should also be supported by the examinee with some prior knowledge or personal beliefs.

The Paper-based Test (PBT)

This type of test is taken in place of the Internet-based test in some areas where Internet access is not available. Registration for the PBT can be done online, or by submitting a registration form that is provided in the Supplemental Paper TOEFL Bulletin. This type of test is given six times annually, so advanced registration is recommended to avoid running out of seats. There are limited number of seats so be prompt in registration (About the TOEFL® PBT Test, 2010).

You can take all the test sections on the same day. It can be also taken as many times as you want, but the most recent score is the one which is considered.

• Listening

Description: Part 1: 30 questions about a brief conversation

Part 2: 8 questions about longer conversations

Part 3: 12 questions about lectures or discussions

Testing Time: 30-40 minutes

Total Questions: approx. 50

• Structure and Written Expression

Description: Consists of items that requires to complete sentences correctly and error identification

Testing Time: 25 minutes

Total Questions: 40 (15 sentence completion, 25 error identification)

• Reading Comprehension

Description: Consists of reading passages

Testing Time: 55 minutes

Total Questions: 50 questions

• **Writing**

Description: Requires writing an essay

Testing Time: 30 minutes

Total Questions: 1

The final scores for Paper-based tests have the range of 310-677 points. That is based on three sub scores.

> Listening (31-68)
>
> Structure (31-68)
>
> Reading (31-67)

The examinees' scores are not determined by the percentage of their correct answers. This is because some tests are more difficult than the others. The scores are converted to a different scoring system to be fair in rating.

Tips on How to Ace TOEFL Exams

English may be your secondary or tertiary language, and you may think it will not be necessary to be fluent in it. But since you plan to work in an English-speaking country like the Unites States, you have no choice but to adapt a foreign tongue. Taking the TOEFL can be very difficult because it measures all the language proficiency skills. If you want to improve your English, try the following suggestions.

1.   Watch English movies or TV shows. You will learn new words and the right pronunciation of words you are not familiar with.

2.   Read English books. Whether it is fiction or non-fiction, for academic reasons or entertainment, it will help you in improving your grammar and broadening your vocabulary.

3.   Listen to English songs. It may sound crazy, but since most popular songs have

English lyrics, you have the tendency to memorize the song and it can also help you build up your vocabulary.

4.   Talk to English-speaking people. If you happen to know someone who is from an English speaking country, why not strike a conversation with him or her? This can be awkward for you, but this will also serve as a sort of training.

5.   Consult a dictionary when you encounter a word you are not familiar with. If you can, list the words you don't know that you encounter, while reading or watching TV. This will broaden your vocabulary.

Test of Spoken English

As of March 31, 2010, the Test of Spoken English was cancelled. See ETS' website for more updates (www.ets.org/tse). The Test of Spoken English (TSE) measures nonnative English speakers' oral communication skills. In this test, you will demonstrate your oral communication ability in English through oral response, under timed conditions. This tests your comprehension in oral communication setting and also your fluency in spoken English.

Test of Written English

The Test of Written English (TWE) is a component of the Test of English as a Foreign Language (TOEFL). It determines the writing ability of nonnative English speakers. It also evaluates the proficiency of individuals in reading and writing English. As a physical therapist, being proficient in written English may not be of utmost importance, but since comprehension and articulation of ideas are important to communicate effectively, it must not be disregarded.

This type of test requires the examinee to write an essay about a brief topic. Examinees then organize and relate their thoughts about the given topic. The scoring system ranges for 1 to 6, with 6 being the highest (Test of Written English Guide, 2004).

Scores are determined by some of these criteria:

- Topic is addressed properly

- Organization of ideas

- Development of ideas

- Clarity

- Appropriate details supporting the ideas

- Consistent facility in using English

- Syntactic variety

- Appropriate use of words

- Quality of essay

Examinees would be asked to give reaction, explanation, or ideas about a statement or statements.

Tips in answering TWE Questions

1.   Read the topic carefully. Take time to understand what it asks for. If it asks to discuss your side on a certain issue, then you should relate your position on that issue. Don't stray away from the topic.

2.   There is space provided for your notes. It is better if you outline your essay before you finally write it down. You may write down notes, phrases or ideas on this space to make it easier for you to organize your ideas.

3.   Express your ideas clearly. Don't be too wordy or use words that may not be appropriate for an idea. For example, the words "ensure-- insure" and "complimentary—complementary". The word ensure signifies guaranteeing something, while insure simply means buying an insurance policy for something such as a car, or a house. Complementary refers to something that completes another thing, while the word complimentary describes

something which is given as an incentive or praise. These two words should not be used in place of one another.

4.   Writing a very long essay will not guarantee a good score. Quality is more emphasized by this type of test.

5.   If you can, add details to support your statements. Just make sure that these details are relevant to the topic.

6.   Always check your sentence construction.

7.   You have 30 minutes to finish the TWE. Express your opinions effectively using brief and clear sentences.

8.   If you have finished your essay ahead of time, you can revise and check your work.

9.   If the time is already up, stop writing. If you don't, it is already considered as a form of cheating.

Alternate Identification Number
A Substitute for a U.S. Social Security number?

There are cases when a candidate for NPTE cannot obtain a Social Security number. There might be some problems with his or her application, or the candidate has not yet received his or her SSN by the time he or she is going to take the NPTE. Social Security number is a requirement for taking the NPTE. An "Alternate Identification Number" is given by the FSBPT for a candidate with no Social Security Number yet. This can be obtained through application. You can find the application form for AIN at FSBPT's website. Go to this link www.fsbpt.org/NPTE/AINApp.

The Alternate Identification Number only serves the purpose of registering for examinations or services through the FSBPT. The AIN is not a substitute for a Social Security Number. You cannot use the AIN to open a bank account or to get a driver's license.

Applicants should retain their AIN and utilize it concerning all correspondence, inquiries, or requests relating to their licensure examination. Completed forms should be mailed to FSBPT, Exam Services, 124 West Street South, 3rd Floor, Alexandria, Virginia 22314. (Alternate identification number, a substitute for a U.S. social security number?, 2008)

Licensing

The Application Process

It is important that you have prepared all your important documents before applying as a physical therapist in the United States. Below are some documents you need to prepare:

- Authentic Birth Certificate

- Passport

- Transcript of Records (from college)

- Police Clearance

- References from companies/facilities you have worked for

You may not need all of these in your application process, but it is best you have them all at hand just in case the employer/agency asks for these documents. If you have prepared all your important documents in advance, you will find the application process easy.

1. Finding an Employer to Sponsor You

There are many agencies, hospitals and clinics looking for foreign-educated physical therapists. You can find them in newspaper ads, the Internet or by referral. The agency you are applying for could be a local or a U.S.-based agency. If you are applying to a local agency, be sure to check the eligibility of that agency. You can ask local government agencies responsible for foreign employment matters about an agency's eligibility. Taking this step will help you avoid illegal recruiters that will just take advantage of you. (See Choosing a Sponsoring Agency for more information).

2. Sending Your Resume

Once you have found an agency, send your resume/curriculum vitae to them. In your objectives, indicate the state where you want to work. An agency may look through your experience as a physical therapist, but fresh graduates don't have to worry as long as they have passed local licensure examinations and had a record of good academic performance. Another thing agencies consider is an applicant's fluency in English. Your resume reflects this, so before sending them your resume, check for spelling and grammatical errors.

3. Interview

The interview is usually done by phone, if you are still in your native country. But if you are already in the U.S., it is best if you are interviewed personally.

4. Signing a Contract

If your application is already approved, the agency will offer you a written contract. That contract contains all terms and conditions, services and fees for the rest of the process. Read the contract carefully before you sign it. If you can, get expert advice, ideally from a lawyer. This is advised if you find some things in the contract which confuses you.

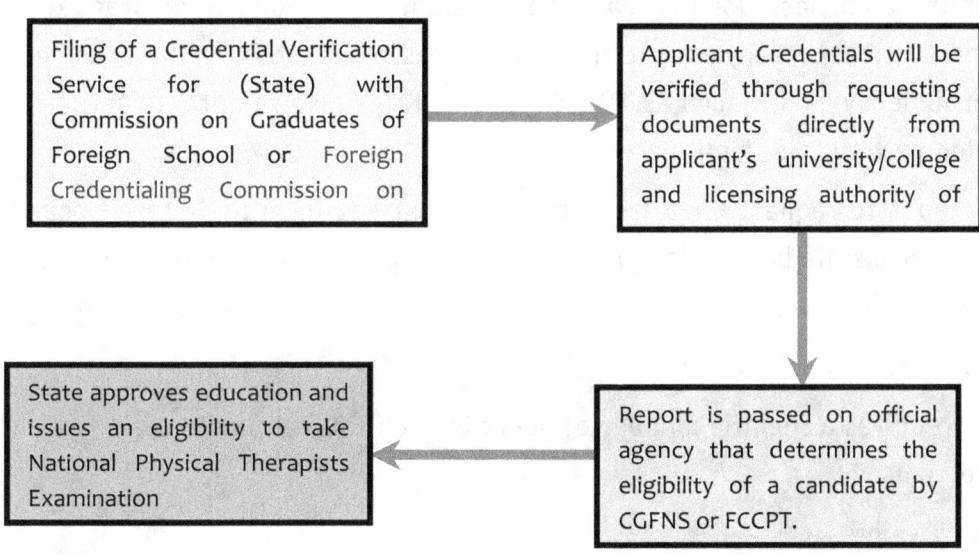

5.   Agreement

Upon signing the contract, you and the employer has agreed on matters concerning your work and their fees. The agency you applied to will take charge of your visa/green card application.

*Note: This process may not apply to all states; each state has its own licensing procedures.

6.   Agency Sponsors Applicant Visa

The agency will then sponsor the foreign educated physical therapist applicant for a visa. They will decide which kind of visa, if it is H1B or a green card. After getting your H1B or green card, you can now work in a facility where your agency will places you (Physical Therapists-The Process, n.d.).

Getting a License Without a Sponsoring Agency

1.   You have to get a license to practice your profession in the US. First thing you do is to choose a prospective state where you want to practice. This is to determine the state's specific requirements, since requirements vary in each state. Each state also works with specific credentialing agencies. Usually, each state requires the following: graduation from an accredited physical therapy education program; passing the NPTE; jurisprudence exams; English proficiency exams such as TOEFL. Some states also require a continuous study as a condition to maintain license.

2.   The next step is to request for a free application packet from that state's board. Contact your prospective state board. Below is a list of things you have to consider because they vary by state:

•   Credentialing agency

Each state requires a specific number of hours in each subject plus the breakdown of clinical requirements.

•   Proficiency Exams

These proficiency exams determine a foreign physical therapists' command in English. These are the TOEFL (Test of English as Foreign Language), TSE and TWE. Some states may not require them at all.

• Visa Screen Certificate Requirement

You can check these two sources:

www.cgfns.org

www.fccpt.org

3. The next thing to do is to apply for an alternate identification number (AIN). This is processed in a period of five (5) days after receipt. This is issued by the FSBPT when a candidate cannot get a Social Security Number.

4. After the application is completed, it should be mailed to FSBPT. The purpose of issuing an AIN is to let a candidate register for examinations and services through FSBPT if a Social Security Number cannot be released for that candidate.

5. Then, you have to contact FSBPT for exam registration. Once verified, an authorization to take the test will be mailed to you. This authorization is valid for 60 days.

6. The next step is to contact Prometric for an examination schedule. The exam can only be taken within the United States. You have to obtain an appropriate visa before you can go to the United States to take the exam. These visas are granted by the United States Citizenship and Immigration Services. You should have an appointment for your application. You may opt to apply for a tourist visa first, if you are intending to take the NPTE only.

You can call the USCIS National Customer Service Center (NCSC) at 1-800-375-5283 (TTY 1-800-767-1833) if you have any question with regards to immigration procedures or any clarification. This call center is toll free, and live assistance may be available in English or Spanish. The National Customer Service Center will only provide answers to your queries, but not any updates or information about your case status.

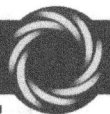

Credentialing Agencies

Physical Therapy curriculum varies from country to country. Each country has its own educational system. To make sure that your physical therapy education is equivalent to the US standard, you have to get a credential evaluation from credentialing agencies. This will verify if the program you have attended meets the American Physical Therapists Association standards, and will also determine if your college or university is APTA accredited. This is important because you have to prove educational equivalency before you can get a physical therapist license. Before getting any service from any credentialing agencies, make sure that the credentialing agency and the credential evaluation report is approved by your prospective state.

Foreign Credentialing Commission on Physical Therapy (FCCPT)

The Foreign Credentialing Commission on Physical Therapy was created to assess the credentials and qualifications of foreign educated physical therapists. This organization's main goal is to help the United States Citizenship and Immigration Services (USCIS) and jurisdiction licensing authorities by authenticating and verifying the educational and regulatory documents of foreign-trained physical therapists. FCCPT does this by comparing an applicant's educational curriculum through a standard that the Federation of State Boards of Physical Therapy (FSBPT) has developed and validated. The FCCPT is also authorized to do the following:

•   Issuing the required certification of the United States Citizenship and Immigration Services (USCIS)

•   Giving documentation for the Center for Medicare and Medicaid Services (CMS) for foreign physical therapists and PTAs

50 jurisdictions recognize FCCPT to assess educational equivalency for the purpose of

licensure to foreign-trained physical therapists. The New York State for Collection and Verification of documents also recognizes FCCPT for the NY State Education Department review in order to get a license in New York. A number of US educational institutions also recognize FCCPT to provide reports on educational equivalency for admission to an advanced Physical Therapy degree program. The FCCPT also helps foreign physical therapist applicants to identify their deficiencies in their education and fill those by providing opportunities and options (Overview of the Primary Services, n.d.).

The FCCPT offers the following services:

1.   Comprehensive Credential Evaluation Review (Type I Certificate)

This serves individuals who need a Health Care Worker Certificate to get a clearance from the USCIS. This will enable or allow employment in the U.S.. Review Includes:

•   Educational Credentials Review

•   Verification of Eligibility to practice in Country of Education elsewhere if applicable

•   Verification of English Proficiency

•   The Type 1 Certificate is a visa screen and results in (USCIS) Healthcare Worker Certificate

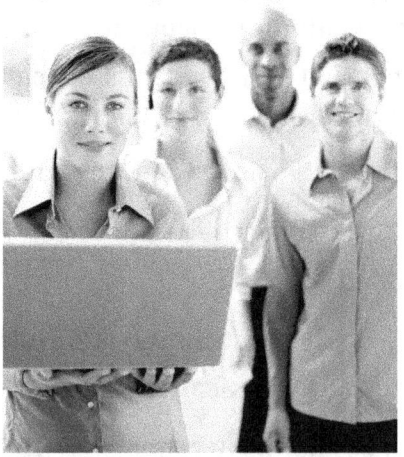

Most states acknowledge the results of the Educational Credentials Review, even though it is just a part of the Type 1 Comprehensive Credential Evaluation for licensure. But it should be noted that some jurisdictions (states) do require the Type I certificate before they process licensure. These jurisdictions include Louisiana, Massachusetts, New Mexico, North Dakota, Tennessee and Washington, D.C.

To be sure, always read the requirements for the jurisdiction you wish to work in to see if they updated their requirements, or any changes have occurred in their requirements list.

How to Get Type I Certificate

1.	Apply and pay for Type I Service online. (Go to www.fccpt.org)

2.	Once you've made a personal account, you can log into your account to view the progress of your application. Be knowledgeable of the items that are required to be sent to the FCCPT.

3.	Send your academic and licensing request forms to their corresponding institutions. These request forms are:

•	Request for Academic Credentials Verification

	Fill out page one, page two will be accomplished by registrar

•	Request for Verification of Physical Therapy License

	Fill out page one, page two will be accomplished by regulatory authority

4.	Submit a signed and notarized Type I attestation page, along with one recent passport size photograph.

5.	Submit a notarized copy of your physical therapy education diploma, degree or certificate. (Marked with "True copy of the original".)

6.	Contact the Educational Testing Services (ETS) and request sending your TOEFL scores to FCCPT (Institution Code of FCCPT: 8164).

7.	Contact the Federation of State Boards of Physical Therapy (FSBPT), request the transfer of your scores to FCCPT (if you have already taken the NPTE).

8.	You can check the progress of your application online anytime when you log in.

9.	You must provide FCCPT with your e-mail address and your mailing address to avoid any problems.

10.   If a third party will be involved, you must submit a notarized release of information, if a third party will contact the FCCPT in your behalf.

THINGS TO REMEMBER:

•   Do not send original copies of your diplomas or certificates. All the documents that you send to FCCPT become their property and they will not return it to you.

•   You are not required to send copies of your transcripts, mark sheets, syllabi and license verifications.

•   Do not forward collected transcripts/verifications in sealed envelopes to FCCPT. This is the job of your academic institution.

The applicant's academic institution should fill out the academic information form and submit it with your full transcripts directly to FCCPT. If it is required, they should also send official course descriptions and/or syllabi to the FCCPT. The documents should be in English, if possible. In case that the documents are in another language, it must be sent along with translations. The academic institution should not send any documents to you or to the translator.

The licensing authority, on the other hand, will fill out the license verification form. The form should be submitted to FCCPT after it is accomplished, and the licensing authority should not send any document to you to forward to FCCPT.

The examining institution's task is to forward your scores on TOEFL, TWE, TSE and IBT to FCCPT. Your NPTE score should be forwarded directly to FCCPT by the FBSPT. Again, the examining institutions should not send the required documents to you. They should send the scores directly to FCCPT. The FCCPT will give you a file number as soon as online payment has been made.

Documents written on your native language will be sent to you upon verification, and you will be instructed to have it translated. FCCPT collects and authenticates all documents as they arrive. There will be an eight week allowance for FCCPT to complete the Type 1 review. After finishing all the reports, FCCPT will send it to you (applicant) and the state (jurisdiction) electronically. Type 1 certificates will be mailed to you after you have met all the requirements.

2.   Visa Credentials Review Service (Type II Certificate)

Foreign physical therapists that have license to work in the U.S. can get a Type II certificate if they can't get a Type I certificate. This is unavailable since September 1, 2009.

3.   Educational Credential Review Service

This credentials review is mainly used for license application to practice physical therapy in the United States. It determines whether the education of a foreign-trained physical therapist matches an accredited physical therapy degree program provided in the United States. This type of review service can also be used for admission into some U.S. educational institutions. It can also be used for CMS certification (for Medicare or Medicaid providers).

4.   New York Verification Process

This service is specifically designed for New York. It is because the New York State Education Department requires this for licensure as Physical Therapists and Physical Therapist Assistants. An independent verification of the validity of one's credentials should be from a NYSED-certified Credential Verification Organization, just like FCCPT.

5.   Planned Learning and Assistance Network

This service helps individuals to identify solutions if they have educational deficiencies (whether their educational program did not pass APTA standards or their program is not accredited) and gives them options to supplement these problems. FCCPT offers this to individuals who subscribed to their services, even those who consulted other review agencies.

The FCCPT does not request your academic, licensing, or examining institutions on (your) behalf of the applicant, they will just contact involved academic institutions, licensing/

registration agencies. The FCCPT does not give a license because it is the job of the jurisdiction board. They are also not responsible for the issuance of a visa, the USCIS does this. A notarized release of information from the applicant is required, in case a third party requests for any specific information.

FCCPT FEE SCHEDULE

FCCPT Comprehensive Credentials Evaluation (Type 1) $750
FCCPT Educational Credentials Review $490
New York Verification Process $390
FCCPT Physical Therapist Assistant Educational Equivalency Review $490
Planned Learning and Assistance Network $450
P-L-A-N increments of ½ hour $100
Reactivation $210
Re-evaluation $350
Type I Certificate Renewal $350
Duplicate Reports $90
Fees for states that require conversion of credentials to a second state $50
Requests for copies for states that require conversion after first review has been compiled and mailed=re-evaluation $350
Photocopies of original documents notarized by FCCPT $25
Change of Service Requests $100
Late Fees $100

   *Fees are subject to change without prior notice.

1.   FCCPT Comprehensive Credentials Evaluation (Type 1) includes certificate and report forwarded to the applicant and a state. A duplicate fee will be charged if additional reports are needed.

2.   The FCCPT Educational Credentials Review includes a review and an additional fee shall be charged for additional reports.

3.   FCCPT Physical Therapist Assistant Educational Equivalency Review includes a report. A Duplicate Report fee shall be collected in case the applicant needs more copies

of the report.

4.   The FULL P-L-A-N counseling includes the cost of one re-evaluation after coursework is completed.

5.   Re-activation fee is charged to an revive expired application.

6.   The basis of re-review evaluation will be the new information that the applicant has provided.

How to apply for a visa, a license and credential review at the same time

The FCCPT suggested some tips on how to apply simultaneously for USCIS, licensure and FCCPT.

•   Choose the state where you want to practice as a physical therapist.

•   Know that state's licensing requirements, application procedures and credentialing agencies that the state approves.

•   Know which types of work visa/permit are needed, then begin to process your visa application with USCIS.

•   Apply to the credentialing agency to see if your education matches the requirements of the jurisdiction you wish to work in.

•   The credentialing agency will forward their final report about your educational evaluation to you and the licensing authority where you want to work in.

•   The licensing authority of that state will review your application for license, which includes your credential evaluation report and they will decide if you are qualified to take the National Physical Therapist Examination (NPTE).

•   Id the state decides that you cannot take the NPTE, you must satisfy their requirements by taking supplemental education. If you have accomplished taking that supplemental education, a re-evaluation of your credentials will be required.

•   If the state/jurisdiction permits you to take the NPTE and you:

Passed - most state boards would issue your license, but some will require a period of supervised practice or acquiring a Social Security Number first before a license is issued.

Failed – a retake will be required, until you earn a passing score.
Contact FCCPT
Foreign Credentialing Commission on Physical Therapy (FCCPT)
511 Wythe Street
Alexandria, VA 22314-1917
Phone 703-684-8406   Fax 703-684-8715   E-mail fccpt@fsbpt.org

Commission on Graduates of Foreign Nursing Schools

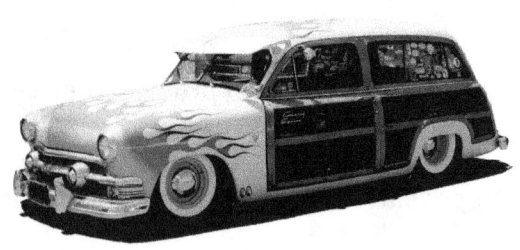

The Commission on Graduates of Foreign Nursing Schools is another credentialing agency which is recognized by most states/ jurisdictions. They offer services similar to FCCPT, but their prices are much lower. It is a globally recognized authority on evaluating academic credentials. CGFNS primarily serves foreign educated/trained nurses, but also serves other health care professions such as physical therapy and non-health care professions worldwide.

Services offered by the Commission on Graduates of Foreign Nursing Schools are:

(List includes services applicable for physical therapists ONLY. Other CGFNS services which are only applicable for nurses or other professions not related to physical therapy are omitted from this list.)

1. Credentials Evaluation Services

The Commission on Graduates of Foreign Nursing Schools International Credentials Evaluation Service is equivalent to FCCPT's Comprehensive Credential Evaluation Review (Type I Certificate)- Educational Credentials Review. The Credentials Evaluation Services (CES) report analyzes the credentials of foreign health care service providers seeking licensure in the U.S. The CES intends to give consultations/advisories, and it does not make placement recommendations (Credentials Evaluation Service, 2010).

CGFNS gives out two kinds of CES Reports:

- Healthcare Profession and Science Report

- Full Education Course-by-Course Report

The result of your CES report is an important tool for regulatory agencies and licensing agencies as well. It is also valuable to specialty certification authorities, academic institutions, immigration attorneys and foreign trained physical therapists employers. This also validates the merits of an applicant's credentials compared to United States' standards to help foreign educated physical therapists in their pursuit for a career in the United States.

How to apply for a CES Report

1.   Complete the requirements.

- Information about how you discovered the CES and why you chose CGFNS to prepare your credentials report

- Previous Commission on Graduates of Foreign Nursing Schools/ International Commission on Healthcare Professions (CGFNS/ICHP) application, state/jurisdiction where you want to practice, country where you have worked, your nature of work, years you spent on that work

- The **name** you want to appear on your Credentials Evaluation Service Report. Also supply all the names you have used in the past (for example, you have your name changed due to a mistake in spelling, variations of your name, surname...) This is for CGFNS to easily recognize your documents. Also include legal documents and notarized affidavits about your change of name. If married, also attach a marriage certificate or notarized affidavit.

• **Residence address** (where you live) and mailing address (where you want to receive mails from CGFNS). If you change any of these addresses, you must contact CGFNS at once.

• **Marital status information**, if married, be sure to have your marriage certificate at hand.

• **Birth Date**-should be entered as (month-day-year) where the month is spelled out.

• **Gender and citizenship** (take note, citizenship is different from nationality for example, you may be of Chinese descent but a Korean citizen), native language. Provide citizenship identification number if applicable.

• **Contact Details** – telephone number, mobile (cell phone) number, fax number and e-mail address.

• **U.S. Social Security Number**

• **Education** – all information about your primary, secondary and professional healthcare educational institutions you have attended should be listed down, along with dates. Send a copy of the "Request for Academic Records" to each school you have attended. CGFNS only accepts documents coming directly from the educational institution.

2. You can apply online or by mail

• Online Application

   Create a CGFNS Connect Account to order service

   Submit order service

• Mail application

CGFNS-CREDENTIALS EVALUATION SERVICES FEES

ONLINE APPLICATION/PAPER APPLICATION

Full Education Course-By-Course Report application	$385.00	/$460.00
Healthcare Profession & Science Report application	$335.00	/$410.00
Reprocess a Full Education Course-By-Course Report application	$150.00	/$225.00
Reprocess a Healthcare Profession & Science Report application	$125.00	/$200.00
Additional CES report recipients	$ 60.00	/$60.00
Evaluation of additional academic credential	$60.00	/$60.00
Evaluation of additional registration/license	$60.00	/$60.00
Duplicate Credentials Evaluation Service report for applicant	$60.00	/$60.00
Re-evaluation of a Full Education Course-by-Course Report	$250.00	/$325.00
Re-evaluation of a Healthcare Profession & Science Report	$195.00	/$270.00

*Fees are subject to change without prior notice.

Reprocessing of report applications (Full Education Course-by-Course & Healthcare Profession & Science Report) are for those applicants who have already paid in full, but have not completed the requirements in twelve (12) months. The reprocessing is accepted after the expiration of the first Full Education Course-By-Course Report application or Healthcare Profession & Science Report application.

2.   Credential Verification Service (CVS) for New York State

This credential verification service is specialized for the state of New York. CGFNS sends a report to the New York State Education Department. The authentication of your official documents is the main purpose of this service. It does not analyze or determine if your education is enough. It does not give recommendations regarding your eligibility for a license in the state of New York. You can have your credentials evaluated separately by the New York State Education Department and you have to send the forms to them, and not to CGFNS. You will not be furnished with a copy of the report that will be sent to the New York State Education Department. You can check your status on the CGFNS website. "Report Issued" will be displayed on your status once the report has been sent to the New York State Education Department.

The New York State Education Department will be the one to contact you with regard to your eligibility.

How to apply for CVS for New York State?

You can apply online or by mail. Log on to cgfns.org

LIST OF SERVICES

ONLINE APPLICATION	/PAPER APPLICATION	
Credential Verification Service of New York State application	$390.00	/$465.00
Reapplication	$390.00	/$465.00
Re-issue report	$ 75.00	/$ 75.00

*Fees are subject to change without prior notice.

3. VisaScreen®: Visa Credentials Assessment

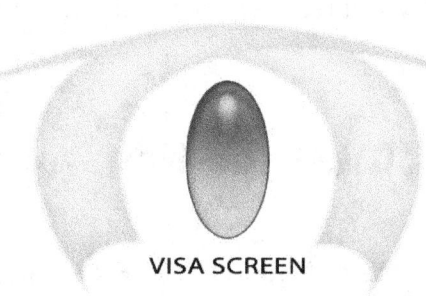

VISA SCREEN

As stated on the Illegal Immigration Reform and Immigrant Responsibility Act (IIRIRA, 1996) Section 343, specific healthcare professionals, including physical therapists are required to complete a screening program. That is prior to their acquisition of a permanent or temporary occupational visa. This also includes the Trade NAFTA status. This VisaScreen® contains an evaluation of the applicant's education, compared to U.S. standards, authentication of professional health care licenses and an English proficiency exam.

Upon accomplishing VisaScreen®, you will receive an International Commission on Healthcare Professions VisaScreen® certificate, one of the Federal screening requirements.

VISASCREEN SERVICES
ONLINE APPLICATION   /PAPER APPLICATION

	ONLINE APPLICATION	PAPER APPLICATION
VisaScreen® application (Valid for 5 years)	$540.00	/$615.00
Reprocess an expired application	$150.00	/$225.00
VisaScreen®: Expedited Review Service	$500.00	/$500.00
Application for renewal certificate	$275.00	/$350.00
Certificate verification letter	$100.00	/$100.00
Replacement certificate (limit 1)	$150.00	/$150.00

*Fees are subject to change without prior notice.

All applicants would be given a 12-month period to complete all the requirements of the application order. If a fully paid application has expired, the applicant is given another 12 months to reprocess his or her application.

International Credentialing Associates

Another credentialing agency is the International Credentialing Associates. They provide educational credential evaluation reports to government agencies, immigration attorneys etc. Their physical therapy evaluations list relevant coursework on specific Board-designated forms. They also list proprietary FCCPT Coursework Tools, which is a copyright of the Federation of State Boards of Physical Therapy (Welcome, 2010).

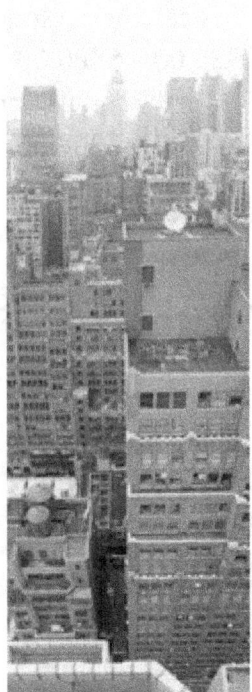

Contact ICA: International Credentialing Associates
7245 Bryan Dairy Road
Bryan Dairy Business Park II
Largo, FL 33777
Phone: (727)549-8555
Fax: (727)549-8554

Processing Time: 12 weeks

Fees: $425

International Consultants of Delaware, Inc.

The International Consultants of Delaware Inc. also provides Physical Therapy and Physical Therapy Assistant Credentials Evaluations. Their evaluation can be used for applying for state board licensure in the United States. Their PT and PTA Credentials Evaluations contain: Duration of Study, List of Institutions, Degrees/Diplomas/Certificates earned, Comparison of International educational credentials to US, licensure in the country of origin, total number of educational credits earned, sources of educational credentials including transcripts, diplomas, degrees, certificates (submitted directly to ICD) and lastly, state board form which enlists categories/courses/credits for certain state boards of physical therapy.

ICD Fees Schedule

Credentials Evaluation Services

Physical Therapist /Physical Therapy Assistant

Physical Therapist and Physical Therapy Assistant Report (2009 varies by state)

$325.00 – $500.00   /$75.00 – $170.00

Physical Therapist and Physical Therapy Assistant Report (2010 varies by state)

$400.00 – $500.00   /$75.00 – $170.00

Re-evaluation Report (to have additional credentials evaluated toward your original application)

FULL FEE

States that Recognize ICD Credentials Evaluation

- ❑ Alaska
- ❑ Arizona
- ❑ Arkansas
- ❑ California
- ❑ Colorado
- ❑ Delaware
- ❑ Florida
- ❑ Guam
- ❑ Hawaii

- ❑ Idaho
- ❑ Indiana
- ❑ Iowa
- ❑ Kansas
- ❑ Kentucky
- ❑ Maine
- ❑ Maryland
- ❑ Michigan

❏ Minnesota		❏	Puerto Rico
❏ Missouri		❏	South Carolina
❏ Montana		❏	South Dakota
❏ Nebraska		❏	Virgin Islands
❏ New Jersey		❏	Virginia
❏ New Mexico		❏	Washington
❏ North Carolina		❏	Wisconsin
❏ Ohio		❏	Wyoming

Note: Contact the state board of your prospective state first before deciding what kind of evaluation report they are requiring. Also, the list above is subject to change without prior notice.

Processing Time: 14 days

(ICD Physical Therapy and Physical Therapy Assistant Credentials Evaluations for applicants educated outside the United States, 2010)

Contact ICD:

International Consultants of Delaware, Inc

P.O. Box 8629
Philadelphia, PA 19101-8629
TEL: (215) 222-8454 ext. 510
FAX: (215) 349-0026
Web site: www.icdel.com
E-mail: icd@icdel.com

Educational Credentials Evaluators

The Educational Credential Evaluators, Inc. (ECE) also provides evaluation reports that compare the U.S. equivalents of educational qualifications earned by foreign trained physical therapists. (Frequently Asked Questions, n.d.)

ECE offers different types of evaluation reports:

REPORTS	FEES
General	$85
Course-by-Course	$135
Subject Analysis	$ 175
Catalog Match	$ 225
Health Professions Licensure	$ 250

Before you decide which report you will subscribe to, contact the state board of the jurisdiction you will apply to first.

Processing Time: 1, 5,-12 business days (depending on the report)

Contact ECE:

Educational Credential Evaluators, Inc.

PO Box 514070

Milwaukee WI 53203-3470 USA

414-289-3400 | eval@ece.org

Credentialing Problems

If you have deficiencies in your credits, here are the following things you can do:

1.   Talk to the credentialing agency. Ask them what you can do so that you can be at par with the U.S. standard. Usually, credentialing agencies have suggestions such as taking a continuing education course, taking an online course, going back to college (we hope you will not resort to this) and so forth...

2.   Contact your school to provide evidence to prove that this deficiency was taken as part of your school's PT course. There are two types of deficiencies: a.) You do not have enough credit units. b.) You did not have supporting documents to prove that you indeed took the course. Your school can help you in both situations.

For example, your credentialing report states that you only have 67 professional units and you lack geriatric rehabilitation.

The state you are applying for requires 69 professional units. As you were reading your report, you noticed that they did not credit you for undergraduate thesis, a 3-credit course. You can ask your school to provide them a letter that your undergraduate thesis is equivalent to a U.S. course called Research Methods. Assuming a multiplying factor of 1 foreign credit is to 0.75 U.S. credit, you will gain 2.25 credits on your credentialing report. This will raise your units into 69.25.

How about the deficient course? As with the example above, the credentialing agency did not credit you for geriatric rehabilitation. You know very well that you took this course in one of your subjects but with a different name. Maybe, you took it on Medical-Surgical Lectures? Medical Rehabilitation Lectures? Theory and Technique? It is up to you. You try to think clearly which subject you took geriatric rehabilitation and ask your school to provide evidence that this subject is indeed taken on a particular course with a different name.

3.   Contact your state board. You have contacted your school and you still have a few subjects deficient... You contacted the credentialing agency and they said that they have reviewed the additional documentation you have provided, however, it is still not at par with the U.S. standard. The next step is to contact the state board.

For example, the credentialing report states that you lack wound debridement (integumentary rehabilitation) and pharmacology. You are sure that you did not take this course on your undergraduate degree. Ask them if you can take a continuing education course, or an online course. Some state boards will allow you to take a continuing education course. This is very helpful when you are in the U.S. There are a lot of wound debridement courses around. Also, there is a lot of online continuing education available. For example, AT Still University caters to students applying for a physical therapy license who lack some credits. The courses taken in AT Still University are purely online. You can easily take a pharmacology course with them and finish it in 6 weeks.

Remember! Before you take any course, be sure to check with the state board first. They will ultimately decide if they will accept an online course or not. There are times that credentialing agencies won't accept a course but the state board will. Follow the state board, they have the authority to grant you the physical therapy license (Credentialing Problems, 2008).

College Level Examination Program (CLEP) for Physical Therapists with Deficiencies in General Education Courses

The College-Level Examination Program® (CLEP) gives you the opportunity to receive college credit for what you already know by earning qualifying scores on any of 34 examinations. Earn credit for knowledge you've acquired through independent study, prior course work, on-the-job training, professional development, cultural pursuits, or internships.

The cost of a CLEP exam is $65, a fraction of the tuition and fees for the corresponding course. Most colleges and universities grant credit for CLEP exams, but not all. There are 2,900 institutions that grant credit for CLEP and each of them sets its own CLEP policy. In other words, each institution determines for which exams credit is awarded, the scores required and how much credit will be granted. Therefore, before you take a CLEP exam, check directly with the college or university you plan to attend.

Not all colleges award the same amount of CLEP credit for individual tests. Furthermore, some colleges place a limit on the total amount of credit you can earn through CLEP or other exams. Other colleges may grant you exemption but no credit toward your degree. Knowing several colleges' policies concerning these issues may help you decide which college to attend. If you think you can pass a number of CLEP exams, you may want to attend a college that will allow you to earn credit for all or most of them.

The College-Level Examination Program has a policy that candidates may not repeat a CLEP exam of the same title within six months. Scores of exams repeated earlier than six months will be canceled and test fees forfeited.

Colleges usually award CLEP credit only to their enrolled students. There are other stipulations, however, that vary from college to college. CLEP exams are administered at approximately 1,300 test centers located on college campuses across the United States and around the world. Find one near you using the CLEP Test Centers search. Then, contact the test center directly to find out its registration procedure. Be sure to ask about its service fee and testing schedule, and parking/transportation information.

Editor's note:

CLEP is useful when you are already here in the United States since most of the courses here cost a lot more than $65. However, if you are still in your country, a good option will be to study at your local accredited college to make up for these deficiencies.

CLEP testing centers are located all over the world. Visit their website for more details at www.collegeboard.com.

Reference:
College-Level Examination Program (CLEP)
P.O. Box 6600
Princeton, NJ 08541-6600
Phone: (800) 257-9558
Fax: (609) 771-7088
Email: clep@info.collegeboard.org

PTSponsor.com does not warrant the accuracy or validity of the information and hereby disclaims any liability to any person for any loss or damage caused by errors or omissions in the site. PTSponsor.com also is not responsible for any material or information contained in the linked sites provided. The information presented at this site should not be construed to be formal legal advice or the formation of any relationship (College Level Examination Program, 2008).

H-1B Visa for Physical Therapists

Specialty workers (such as Physical Therapists) who want to work in the United States can have permission to work in the U.S. legally by having an H-1B visa, provided that the applicant has at least a bachelor's degree or any equivalent educational attainment to obtain the H-1B visa. The U.S. Congress assigns a quota of 65, 000 H-1B visas per fiscal year. Some employers and employees however, are not subject to this numerical "cap."

After filing Form I-129 (this can be downloaded from USCIS website, uscis.gov), USCIS will send you a receipt. This is to acknowledge that USCIS have received your petition. The USCIS will reject and return your fee or ask for more evidence or information if your petition is found to be incomplete. This will also delay the processing of your petition. The USCIS will notify you, once a decision was made.

If you are in the U.S. in a valid nonimmigrant status, you can begin working for your employer once your Form I-129 is approved. If you are still outside the U.S., your petition will be sent to the U.S. consulate near you. By that time, you can already apply at the U.S. Consulate for a non-immigrant visa. Once the visa is issued, you can now travel to the U.S. and apply for admission.

An employer can also file Form I-907, Request for Premium Processing Service, along with the Form I-129. This is after the employer has received the receipt notice for the Form I-129, at the same USCIS location where it was filed. At first, the period of stay that will be granted to a temporary employee will be up to three years, which can be extended up to six years. The standard processing for the H-1B petition usually takes 3-6 months. For the Premium processing, it only takes about 14 days, that is, if the quota is not yet reached.

Non-immigrant workers who have obtained an H-1B visa can maintain their non-immigrant status, and simultaneously, be beneficiaries of an immigrant visa (green card) petition. The H-1B workers themselves can obtain lawful permanent resident status without affecting their current non-immigrant status.

Students in Optional Practical Training with employers who wish to maintain their employment, as well as any other prospective employee should also begin preparation for any H-1B filing. Copies of diplomas, previous employment letters, and transcripts of courses taken, proof of nonimmigrant status and a detailed resume are some of the documents that will be needed for filing the H-1B package.

Our advice:

1.   Use Overnight Mailing to make sure that application reached USCIS by April 1.

2.   Make sure all requirements and documents are completed before April 1.

3.   Make sure you saved enough money for immigration and licensing. To get an idea of how much the licensing process will cost, visit our expense advisor page athttp://www.ptsponsor.com/expense_adv.php

USCIS Fees (Effective as of May 19, 2010)
*   I 129: Petition for Non-Immigrant Worker - $320.00
*   I-907: Premium Processing Fee - $1,000.00
*   Average Lawyer Fees - $1.000.00- $4,000.00
Additional Fees:
* $1500 for the USCIS Education and Training Fee (if the employer has 25 or more full time employees) or $750 for employers with fewer than 25 full time employees
* $500 for the USCIS anti fraud fee
*   The $500 USCIS Anti Fraud Fee and the $1500 or $750 USCIS Education and Training Fees are not required for H1b renewals/ extensions for the same employer.

"Before contacting the USCIS, USCIS may be able to help you if you have a question about immigration procedures, or need clarification, by calling the USCIS National Customer Service Center (NCSC) at 1-800-375-5283 (TTY 1-800-767-1833). This toll-free call center has additional information and, during their specified office hours, can connect you to live assistance in English and Spanish. The NCSC will be able to answer most questions - although they cannot provide information about the status of your case over the telephone" (H-1B Visa for Physical Therapists, 2010).

Green Card for Physical Therapists

Since the physical therapy profession has been designated by the U.S. Department of Labor to be a Schedule A profession, foreign physical therapists are allowed to file for their green cards provided that they have a permanent job offer to work as a physical therapist in the U.S. They should also speak English well, and meet other criteria. They can be enabled to work at any facility in the United States. They wouldn't be forced to work in an area where there is a shortage for physical therapists.

Also, since physical therapy is a Schedule A profession, foreign-trained physical therapists do not have to obtain a Labor Certification from the U.S. Department of Labor (DOL).

The process starts from filing Form I-140 (Immigration Petition for Alien Worker), on behalf of the foreign national with USCIS. A U.S. employer may sponsor a prospective or current foreign national employee. This employee can be inside or outside the U.S. That certain employee should also qualify under one or more of the employment based immigrant visa categories.

In filing a petition, it is shown that the employer and the employee intends to have a professional relationship. Upon the approval of the petition, and there is proof of the employer-employee relationship and your qualifications, you (the foreign national-employee) will be placed in line among others who are waiting to immigrate. Your qualifications will be based on the same kind of "EB" visa category. If you have reached your place in the waiting line, you may be eligible to apply for immigration.

Your place in line, called the "priority date", will be based on the date when your petition was filed with USCIS. It is advantageous to file as early as possible. Because of the high demand and restrictions set by the law on the immigration quota for a fiscal year under each category, waiting periods can vary. Another implication on the waiting periods is the country where you came from. Generally speaking, if a foreign national entered the U.S. legally and is currently in the U.S. (and meets certain other requirements), they may be able to file an application to adjust to permanent resident status if the employment-based

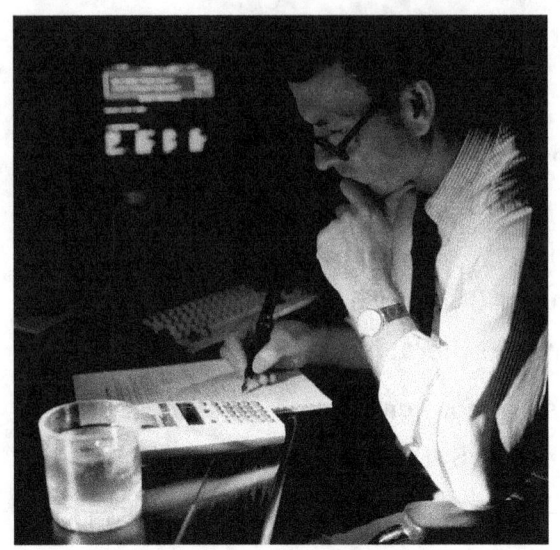

immigrant visa category for that foreign national is "current." And usually, when a foreign national's place in line is reached and their application for immigration is approved, his or her spouse and unmarried children can apply as dependents. Again, the processing time for this depends on various factors.

You can check the current processing times on our website. (http://www.ptsponsor.com/Case_status_online.php)

What is required?

1.   A Physical Therapist with a 4 Year Bachelor Degree in Physical Therapy, or equivalent, and,

2.   A Physical Therapist with a State License, or, A Physical Therapist with a letter from the State Licensing Authority for the state of intended employment stating that the Foreign National Physical Therapist is qualified to take that state's written licensing examination for Physical Therapists.

***If you have a master's degree or higher, file for EB2 instead of EB3. EB2 is for specialized professions with at least a master's degree. The wait for EB2 is usually shorter. Consult an immigration lawyer for details.

Outside the U.S.

The Employer files the Form I-140 and Form ETA 750 with the USCIS. Once the USCIS approves the I-140 Petition, the USCIS first sends the I-140 Petition to the National Visa Center. If there is no backlog for immigrant visas from the Physical Therapist's native country, the Visa Center forwards a packet to the Physical Therapist containing biographical information forms to be completed and a list of documents which must be presented at the interview for permanent residence.

The physical therapist sends the signed and completed forms to the U.S. consulate where the interview for permanent residence will be conducted.

At this interview, the physical therapist must present various documents including the following:

- Application for Immigrant Visa

- Police Clearance

- Birth Certificate

- Marriage Certificate, if any

- Divorce or Death Certificate of Spouse, if any

- Valid Passport

- Medical Examination

- USCIS Photographs

- Recent job offer letter (or employment contract)

- Financial information regarding employer

- Government filing fee

Within the U.S.:

The Employer files the Form I-140 and Form ETA 9089 with the USCIS. The physical therapist may submit an application for Adjustment of Status concurrently with the I-140. The physical therapist may start work as soon as he/she receives Work Authorization. However, a physical therapist cannot qualify for permanent residence until she presents a visa screen certificate issued by the FCCPT/ CGFNS.

Our Advice:

Apply for both H1b and green card for the following reasons:

1.   There are only 65,000 slots available for H1b. If your name was not picked in the lottery, you have to reapply next year. There is no guarantee that your name will be picked the next year either. Having both H1b and green card petitions will guarantee you the soonest possible time to work in the U.S.

2.   If your name gets picked on April 1 (when you are applying for H1b), you can work in the U.S. in October of that year. This working visa is valid for 3 years and is renewable for another 3 more years. Having both H1b and green card provides better options. Once your green card is approved, it allows you to stay in the U.S. for 10 years. Green card is renewable and allows you to apply for citizenship. H1b is fast. Green card allows you to stay in the U.S. longer.

3.   Lastly, H1b requires you to work for the employer who sponsored you. You can only switch employers if the new employer is willing to sponsor you. Also, if you are sponsored as a full time physical therapist, you can only work as a full time physical therapist. Once your green card or your employment authorization is approved, you can work for any employer * and work for any job your heart desires (Green Card for Physical Therapists, 2010).

(*You are required to work for the employer who sponsored you for green card for at least 6 months. This is a requirement set by the USCIS.)
USCIS Fees: (as of May 2010)
•   I-140: Petition for an Immigrant Worker - $475.00
•   I-485: Adjust status and become permanent resident while in the U.S. (includes filing plus biometric - $1,010
•   I-765: Employment Authorization Document - $340.00
Average Lawyer Fees: $2,000-$10,000.00

Social Security Number

Before you can sit for the National Physical Therapy Examination, the FSBPT will require you to provide a unique identification number-the Social Security Number. Some states also require a Social Security number before they issue a license to a foreign trained physical therapist.

What is a Social Security Number?

A Social Security number (SSN) is a nine-digit number that is issued either to U.S. citizens, permanent residents and temporary (working) residents.

The Social Security number is also used as a de facto identification number. When you open a bank account or apply for loans, a Social Security is required (Social Security number, 2010).

Who is responsible for the issuance of a Social Security number?

It is issued by the Social Security Administration. The Social Security Administration is an independent agency of the United States government.

What is the purpose of a Social Security number?

The Social Security number's main purpose is for taxation. It serves as a tracking device for individuals.

How can you get a Social Security number?

You can get a Social Security number by accomplishing Form SS-5 – "Application for a Social Security Number Card." As a general rule, only non-citizens who have permission to work from the Department of Homeland Security (DHS) can apply for a Social Security number.

There is a new process for Social Security Number application as part of the immigration process. This is developed by the Social Security Administration. Foreign physical therapists can now apply for immigrant visas and Social Security number (SSN) cards simultaneously.

How many times can I renew/replace my Social Security card?

You can replace your Social Security card at least three times a year. The limit for replacement is 10 in a lifetime. This is in accordance with the Intelligence Reform and Terrorism Prevention Act.

Applying for a Social Security Number/Card

If you already have applied for an immigrant visa (green card), applying for a social security number is easier. This is because the U.S. government will be using the same information you provided in your immigrant visa application in your Social Security number application. Once you arrive in the United States, all you have to do is to wait for your Social Security number card. This will be mailed to you in the mailing address you have provided. This takes about three (3) weeks.

How is the Social Security Number processed along with your immigrant visa application?

1.   The U.S. Embassy and Consulates in your home country collects information that are necessary for a Social Security number on Form DS-230 (Application for Immigrant Visa and Alien Registration). This is done as part of your immigrant visa process.

2.   While filling up the Form DS-230, you have to answer "YES" on questions 43a and 43b. Question 43a asks you if you would like to be assigned with a Social Security number, which will be given to you by the Social Security Administration. Question 43b asks for your permission for full disclosure of your information to the Immigration and Naturalization Services (INS) and the Social Security Administration (SSA).

3.   The U.S. Embassy and Consulates will send your information to the Department of Homeland Security.

4.   Then, the Department of Homeland Security (DHS) will admit you into the U.S. They will also send your information to the Social Security Administration.

5.   The Social Security Administration will send your Social Security number through mail. Make sure you stay in the mailing address you have provided in your information sheet. In case you have moved, and have not received your Social Security number yet, you have to call the Social Security Administration. You won't have to do this if you already received your Social Security number before you moved (USCIS, 2010).

How much does a Social Security number cost?

The Social Security Administration does not charge any fee for issuance of a Social Security number.

What if I didn't apply for a Social Security number through my visa process?

You must apply for a card at a Social Security Office.

1.   Complete your application form for a Social Security Card (Form SS-5)

2.   Show original documents or copies certified by issuing agency to prove (US citizenship) immigration status:

•   Department of Homeland Security permission to work in the United States

•   Age

•   Identity

•   Immigration Status

3.   Bring or mail complete application and documents to local Social Security office.

Non-U.S. Citizen Accepted Documents

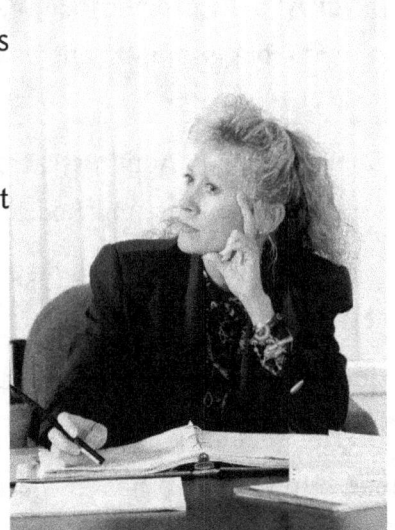

•   Form I-557 (with machine-readable immigrant visa, foreign valid passport)

•   I-94 foreign passport

•   Work permit card from DHS (I-766/I-688B)

Documents to Prove Age

•   Present Birth Certificate

•   Passport

Documents to Prove Identity

•   U.S. Driver's License

- State issued non-driver ID card

- Passport

- Employee ID

- School ID

- Marriage Document

- Health Insurance

- U.S. Military ID

- Adoption Decree

- Life Insurance

Document to Prove Immigration Status

- Any current U.S. Immigration Document

- I-94, Arrival/Departure Record

Note: You should provide original copies of your documents. Certified copies of these documents from issuing agencies are also accepted. Do not send photocopies or notarized copies of documents.

The Social Security Administration issues three types of Social Security card. All of these cards show your name and Social Security number.

1. The first type of card displays your name and SSN. This also lets you work without any restriction.

 The following cards are the so called "restricted" cards.

2. The second type is one which shows your name along with your Social Security number. However, it has a note that says "VALID FOR WORK ONLY WITH DHS AUTHORIZATION."

3. The third type also shows your name and SSN with the note "NOT VALID FOR EMPLOYMENT." (Social Security Number for Non-Citizens or Foreign Workers, 2008).

CHOOSING THE STATE

The following is a list of all U.S. states along with ratings and comments provided by PTSponsor.com and some foreign physical therapists who log in to the site. This should not be your basis of judgment on where you want to work. This will only give you insights about the prospective state you want to work in or provide you information on the most probable conditions you could encounter in that certain state.

We are comparing states based on requirements and ease of obtaining a license. Our top three states are Delaware, New Mexico and New York. All three states do not require the TOEFL. They also allow internationally educated therapists seeking a US license to work with a temporary license for at least six months. Lastly, all three states have no limit in the number of times you can take the exam (in case you fail the first time).

The median hourly wage for the U.S. is $30.33, and the median annual wage is $63,100. In general, the most expensive areas to live are New England, Alaska, Hawaii, and the West Coast. The least expensive continues to be the Midwest and Southern States.

MERIC derives the cost of living index for each state by averaging the indices of participating cities and metropolitan areas in that state. (Bureau of Labor and Statistics. 2007 and Cost of Living, 2007.) ACCRA has changed its name to C2ER. See c2er.org for details and more data products. Cities across the nation participate in ACCRA's survey on a volunteer basis. Price information in the survey is governed by ACCRA collection guidelines which strive for uniformity.

Note: Ratings range from 0-5, with 0 being the lowest and 5, the highest.

ALABAMA

	Therapists' Rating	PTSponsor's Rating
Cost of Living	4	4

License Requirement	1	1
Salary Range	1	4
Overall	2	3

The Good: The cost of living in Alabama is low, and clinical internship is not a requirement.

The Downside: Requirements include English proficiency exams, license from your country of origin and jurisprudence exams. There is also a 3-take limit for the NPTE. They do not offer temporary licenses.

The Bottom Line: Alabama has a lot of requirements. Cost of living is low, while the salary is average.

Other Important Info: Jurisprudence Exam: Required as of May/June 2006; Educational Requirement: 124 semester hours for education completed before 2003; 155 semester hours for education completed 2003 to present; Licensure in Country of Training: Required

ALASKA

	Therapists' Rating	PTSponsor's Rating
Cost of Living	1	1
License Requirement	5	5
Salary Range	5	4
Overall	3.5	2

The Good: Alaska's median annual wage is 78,890. Also, there is no limit on the number of times you take the NPTE.

The Downside: The cost of living here is high. Foreign educated PTs are not given temporary licenses. TOEFL is a requirement.

The Bottom Line: The salary in Alaska is high, however, the requirements and high cost of living must also be considered if you want to work here. Also, the climate is very frigid. Consider the climate here if you can't tolerate low temperatures.

Other Important Info: Application Fee: 50.00, Initial Licensure Fee: 180.00; Total: $230.00; Temporary Licensure for Foreign Trained Therapists: issued when internship is complete without passing the NPTE; 50.00; Clinical Internship: 6 months (preceptor statement); Application process takes 4-6 weeks; Social Security required but may contact board for further details.

ARIZONA

	Therapists' Rating	PTSponsor's Rating
Cost of Living	1	2
License Requirement	2	0
Salary Range	1	4
Overall	1	2

The Good: There is not limit to the number of times you can sit for the NPTE.

The Downside: State does not issue temporary license. 90-day Internship, Jurisprudence and English Proficiency exams are required. The median annual wage is $74, 310, and also, the cost of living is high.

The Bottom Line: Too many requirements and the cost of living is high.

Other Important Info: As of April 1, 2008, the requirement is 90 professional credit hours and 60 general education hours. Deficiencies: college level exam program (CLEP) scores with minimum C can be converted to semester credit hours or college courses; Clinical Internship: 90 days at 40 hours per week, or 180 days at 20 hours per week; You may take the exam twice before having to reapply with a new application and new application fee. FSBPT requires that you submit the exam fee with each and every registration. FSBPT will allow you to retake the exam 3 times within one year beginning with the first exam.; Licensure in Country of Training: Required

ARKANSAS

	Therapists' Rating	PTSponsor's Rating
Cost of Living	4	5
License Requirement	3	2
Salary Range	1	3
Overall	2.5	3

The Good: Arkansas is fourth on the list of states with lowest cost of living.

The Downside: This state does not provide temporary license for Foreign trained PTs, English proficiency exams are also required. If you failed NPTE twice, you have to take a remedial coursework.

The Bottom Line: With a median annual wage of 75,180 and a low cost of living, Arkansas is not a bad place to start.

Other Important Info: Number of times permitted to sit for NPTE: No limit, remedial coursework after 2x; 3 letters of recommendation is required

CALIFORNIA

	Therapists' Rating	PTSponsor's Rating
Cost of Living	1	1
License Requirement	2	0
Salary Range	5	5
Overall	2.5	2

The Good: California ranks second for the highest paying state for PTs. English proficiency exams are not required. There is no limit to the number of times you can take the NPTE.

The Downside: High cost of living neutralizes the high salary. California does not issue a temporary license to foreign PTs. Jurisprudence exams and a 9-month clinical internship are required.

The Bottom Line: Completing all the requirements is worth it because of the generous compensation.

Other Important Info: SSN required. After completion of a deficiency, a new credentialing report is required showing equivalency. They use ELEER (Entry Level Education Equivalency Review). Broken down into: 1955-1978, 1978-1991; 1992-1997;1998-2002; 2003-current; Licensure in Country of Training: Required; Clinical Internship: 9 months; Accepts Joseph Silny and Associates Credentialing

Foreign PTs' Comment: "Tourist Visa won't do. First of all, if you don't have your Social Security Number your application will be returned to you. I know this because my friend already did and her application was returned because PTBC doesn't accept Alternate Identification Number or other Identification Numbers. There are no other exemptions.

You can try to apply to other states first and relocate after a year or once you have your license already in CA. But... If you do have your Social Security Number with you and all the other requirements, PTBC will review your application upon receipt for about 2-3 weeks. Do not contact the board to check on the status of your evaluation. You will receive a letter in the mail, once your credentials have been reviewed."-   A. R.

COLORADO

	PTSponsor's Rating
Cost of Living	3
License Requirement	5
Salary Range	3
Overall	3

The Good: English proficiency exams are not required. There is no limit to the number of times you can sit for the NPTE.

The Downside: The median annual wage in Colorado is one of the lowest, $ 65,780. They do not issue temporary license.

The Bottom Line: The cost of living is Colorado is low. However, the compensation is low.

Other Important Info: Application is on file for 1 year only. Social Security number required but may submit affidavit if you don't have one.

CONNECTICUT

	Therapists' Rating	PTSponsor's Rating
Cost of Living	1	1
License Requirement	3	3
Salary Range	5	5
Overall	3	3

The Good: Connecticut offers a median annual salary of $ 75,420. English proficiency exams are not required.

The Downside: The cost of living is high. They also do not issue temporary licenses.

The Bottom Line: Although the cost of living in Connecticut is high, it has less requirements and offers high salary. It's not a bad place to start.

Other Important Info: 120 hours of college level instruction, 50 hours general education, 60 hours PT education (minimum).

DELAWARE

	Therapists' Rating	PTSponsor's Rating
Cost of Living	4	2
License Requirement	4	5
Salary Range	5	4
Overall	4	4

The Good: Delaware offers a $ 78,040 median annual wage. They also issue temporary licenses. English proficiency exams are not required. There is no limit on the number of times you can take the NPTE.

The Downside: This state has a high cost of living, which makes it a quite expensive place to live in.

The Bottom Line: It has the least number of requirements. Temporary license is valid for 90 days; Temporary license expires upon failure of exam; Applications that are not complete within 6 monthsof filing may be considered abandoned and discarded.

Foreign PTs' Comment: "I'm in Delaware, but they denied me due to short [deficient] in general credits. In the Philippines, we have a 5 year BSPT program. I applied for FCCPT last year. DE needs a minimum of 60 semester credits and 69 semester credits in professional education."- J. T.

DISTRICT OF COLUMBIA

	PTSponsor's Rating
Cost of Living	1
License Requirement	2
Salary Range	3
Overall	2

The Good: License from country of origin and clinical internship are not required.

The Downside: This is an expensive place to live in. English proficiency and jurisprudence exams are required. You can take the NPTE for a maximum of 3x.

The Bottom Line: The median annual wage for D.C. is 78,920. Cost of living and license requirement will make you think twice in choosing this state.

FLORIDA

	Therapists' Rating	PTSponsor's Rating
Cost of Living	1	2
License Requirement	3	2
Salary Range	3	4
Overall	2	3

The Good: Florida has a median annual wage of $ 77,910.

The Downside: Florida ranks 35th on the cost of living list, making it an expensive place to live. Jurisprudence and English proficiency exams are required. Limit for taking exams is five times. In the third attempt, you have to take remedial coursework.

The Bottom Line: The cost of living is high, plus the long list of requirements could be deterrent. The salary is relatively high.

Other Important Info: 5x limit to sit for an exam; **ICD** credentialing fee is $475 (normally $225 for other states); 60 general education credits; 90 professional education credits (67 non-clinical); **CLEP** exam can substitute for general education credits; Social Security required prior to receiving a license.

Foreign PTs' Comment: "They keep your application for 1 year. Fingerprinting is required. You are required to take prevention in medical errors online."- R. M.

GEORGIA

	Therapists' Rating	PTSponsor's Rating
Cost of Living	4	5
License Requirement	1	1
Salary Range	3	4
Overall	2.5	3

The Good: The median annual salary here is $ 74,370. Georgia has a low-cost of living.

The Downside: They do not issue temporary licenses. English proficiency and jurisprudence exams are required. You can only attempt to take the NPTE 4 times, after failing the third attempt, remedial coursework should be taken. You also need a license from the country of training.

The Bottom Line: Although this state requires a lot of documents, the cost of living and salary are worth it.

Other Important Info: 4x limit to sit for an exam; Clinical Internship for 3 months; Application kept on file for 12 months only.

Foreign PTs' Comment: "Bad: SSN required. 3 months of traineeship required. Jurisprudence exam required through FSBPT. You don't get approval for traineeship until board approves all your educational credentials. The board only meets every 2 months. If you send any documents, the website doesn't get updated online until 2-3 weeks. It is a very slow process, especially for the foreign educated. It's very difficult to get in. They accept Physics and Chemistry through CLEP, but re-evaluation is required."- N. N.

HAWAII

	Therapists' Rating	PTSponsor's Rating
Cost of Living	1	1
License Requirement	3	4
Salary Range	1	2
Overall	1.5	2

The Good: Foreign-educated PTs are given temporary licenses. You can sit for NPTE unlimited times.

The Downside: The median annual salary is $ 53,730. Hawaii is one of the most expensive states to live in. TOEFL is a requirement.

The Bottom Line: Although it is one of the states with a least number of requirements, the high cost of living and low salary makes it difficult to practice your profession.

Other Important Info: Temporary license is valid until results of 1st exam. For licensing, social security is required; Application on file for 2 years only.

MAW: Median Annual Wage   MHW: Median hourly wage   JE: Jurisprudence Exam
TL: Temporary License for Foreign Trained PT   NCI: No clinical internship
NNpte: No limit in taking NPTE   SR: Salary Rank (1 highest)   COLAr: Cost of Living Rank (1 highest)

State	MAW	MHW	Credentialing Agency	TOEFL	JE	TL	NCI	NNpte	SR	COLAr
AL	76790	36.92	ICA	YES	YES	NO	NO	YES	24	13
AK	78890	37.93	ICD, FCCPT	YES	NO	YES	YES	NO	6	47
AZ	74310	35.73	ICA, ICD, FCCPT	YES	YES	NO	YES	YES	31	36
AR	75180	36.14	ICA, ICD, IERF, FCCPT	YES	YES	NO	NO	YES	30	9
CA	81530	39.2	ICA, ICD, FCCPT	YES	YES	NO	YES	NO	2	49
CO	65780	31.62	ICA, ICD, FCCPT	NO	NO	NO	NO	NO	45	31
CT	75420	36.26	FCCPT	NO	NO	NO	NO	NO	5	46
DC	78040	37.52	ICD, IERF, FCCPT	NO	NO	YES	NO	NO	14	30
DE	78920	37.94	FCCPT	YES	YES	NO	NO	YES	27	50
FL	77910	37.46	ICD, FCCPT	YES	NO	NO	NO	YES	12	35
GA	74370	35.75	ICA, IERF, FCCPT	YES	YES	NO	YES	YES	18	11
HI	53730	25.83	ICA, ICD, IERF, FCCPT	YES	NO	YES	NO	NO	38	51
ID	69280	33.31	ICA,ICD,IERF,FCCPT	NO	NO	NO	NO	YES	32	10
IL	79640	38.29	FCCPT	YES	NO	NO	NO	NO	22	24
IN	70380	33.84	ICA,ICD,FCCPT	NO	NO	YES	NO	YES	26	12
IA	68980	33.17	FCCPT	YES	NO	NO	NO	NO	37	16
KS	71500	34.37	ICA,ICD,IERF,FCCPT	YES	NO	NO	NO	NO	39	6
KY	73130	35.16	ICD,IERF,FCCPT	YES	YES	YES	YES	NO	28	15
LA	75840	36.46	FCCPT	YES	NO	YES	YES	NO	3	19
ME	65610	31.54	FCCPT	YES	NO	NO	YES	YES	46	37
MD	85770	41.24	ICA,ICD,IERF,FCCPT	YES	YES	YES	NO	NO	7	44
MA	73470	35.32	FCCPT	NO	NO	NO	NO	NO	23	43
MI	73500	35.34	ICD,IERF	YES	YES	NO	NO	NO	8	25
MN	69240	33.29	FCCPT	YES	NO	YES	YES	NO	40	32
MS	71830	34.53	FCCPT	YES	NO	NO	NO	YES	34	7
MO	65210	31.35	FCCPT	YES	NO	YES	NO	YES	40	5

State	MAW	MHW	Credentialing Agency	TOEFL	JE	TL	NCI	NNpte	SR	COLAr
MT	60550	29.11	ICA,FCCPT	YES	YES	YES	NO	YES	43	34
NE	68050	32.72	ICA,ICD,IERF,FCCPT	YES	YES	YES	NO	NO	21	8
NV	80110	38.52	FCCPT	YES	NO	NO	YES	NO	4	38
NH	69100	33.22	FCCPT	YES	NO	NO	NO	NO	42	39
NJ	82110	39.48	ICA,ICD,IERF,FCCPT	YES	YES	NO	NO	NO	1	45
NM	64750	31.13	ICA,ICD,FCCPT	NO	YES	YES	NO	YES	41	29
NY	71420	34.34	FCCPT	NO	NO	YES	NO	NO	25	48
NC	74480	35.81	ICA,ICD,IERF,FCCPT	YES	NO	NO	NO	NO	17	18
ND	64760	31.14	FCCPT	YES	YES	NO	YES	NO	47	21
OH	74390	35.76	ICD,IERF,FCCPT	YES	YES	NO	NO	NO	9	17
OK	67000	32.21	FCCPT	YES	NO	YES	YES	YES	19	4
OR	73580	35.38	IERF,FCCPT	YES	YES	YES	NO	YES	12	41
PA	72090	34.66	FCCPT	NO	NO	NO	YES	YES	15	27
RI	77420	37.22	FCCPT	NO	NO	NO	NO	NO	29	42
SC	71340	34.3	ICD,IERF,FCCPT	YES	NO	NO	YES	YES	36	14
SD	65420	31.45	FCCPT	YES	NO	NO	NO	NO	44	2
TN	75230	36.17	FCCPT	YES	NO	NO	YES	NO	10	1
TX	78770	37.87	ICA,ICD	YES	YES	YES	NO	YES	5	3
UT	67940	32.67	FCCPT	NO	YES	NO	NO	NO	33	20
VT	64510	31.01	ICA,FCCPT	NO	NO	YES	NO	NO	48	40
VA	75520	36.31	FCCPT	YES	NO	YES	YES	NO	13	26
WA	72640	34.92	ICA,ICD,IERF,FCCPT	YES	YES	NO	NO	YES	16	33
WV	74800	35.96	ICA	YES	NO	YES	YES	NO	11	22
WI	72570	34.89	ICA,ICD,IERF,FCCPT	YES	YES	YES	NO	NO	20	23
WY	70360	33.83	IERF,FCCPT	YES	NO	NO	NO	YES	35	28

MAW: Median Annual Wage   MHW: Median hourly wage   JE: Jurisprudence Exam
TL: Temporary License for Foreign Trained PT   NCI: No clinical internship
NNpte: No limit in taking NPTE   SR: Salary Rank (1 highest)   COLAr: Cost of Living Rank (1 highest)

IDAHO

	PTSponsor's Rating
Cost of Living	3
License Requirement	3
Salary Range	3
Overall	3

The Good: English proficiency and jurisprudence exams are not included in their requirements.

The Downside: The median annual wage is $ 69,280. Temporary licenses are not issued. You can only take the NPTE up to 3x; you have to take remedial coursework after the second failed attempt.

The Bottom Line: Idaho has an average cost of living. Application fees consist of: Application-$50, License-$65, Exam Administration- $ 40.

Other Important Info: 3x limit to sit for the NPTE; after 2x, you are required to take remedial coursework; Application on file for 3 years.

ILLINOIS

	Therapists' Rating	PTSponsor's Rating
Cost of Living	3	3
License Requirement	2	2
Salary Range	3	5
Overall	2.5	3

The Good: There is no limit on the number of times you can take the NPTE. But on the third failed attempt, you have to take remedial coursework.

The Downside: Does not issue temporary license. English proficiency exams are required.

The Bottom Line: The cost of living in Illinois is average. The salary and requirements are also average. Application fees include: Acceptance of Exam-$100, Application-$86.50, Licensure-$100

Other Important Info: No limit to sit for the NPTE, however, after failing 3x, you are required to take remedial coursework.

Foreign PTs' Comment: "I studied physical therapy in the Philippines. Illinois accepts a waiver from school stating that English was the medium of instruction used."- M. G.

INDIANA

	PTSponsor's Rating
Cost of Living	4
License Requirement	2
Salary Range	4
Overall	3

The Good: Indiana is a relatively inexpensive place to live in. English proficiency exams are not required.

The Downside: They do not issue temporary licenses. The limit for taking the NPTE is up to three times only.

The Bottom Line: The median annual wage here is $ 70,380. In terms of salary and license requirements, this state is average. The low cost of living is one of its advantages. Social Security Number is mandatory. Without SSN, application will not be processed.

IOWA

	PTSponsor's Rating
Cost of Living	4
License Requirement	0
Salary Range	3

Overall	2

The Good: The cost of living in Iowa is low.

The Downside: Iowa's median annual wage is $68,980. There is no limit to the number of times you can take the exam. However, you must take remedial coursework after failing the exam for 3 consecutive times. TOEFL is required. Foreign trained therapists are not issued a temporary license.

The Bottom Line: The cost of living and salary are both low. No limit to sit for the NPTE, however, after failing 3x, you are required to take remedial coursework.

KANSAS

	PTSponsor's Rating
Cost of Living	4
License Requirement	2
Salary Range	3
Overall	3

The Good: The cost of living in Kansas is average, it ranked 20th.

The Downside: The salary is low, at $71,500. They do not issue temporary licenses. There is no limit on the times you can take the NPTE, but if you have failed three times, you will be required to take a remedial coursework. TOEFL is required.

The Bottom Line: Although the cost of living is low, the requirements are numerous and the salary is low.

Other Important Info: No limit to sit for the NPTE, however, after failing 3x, you are required to take remedial coursework; ICD credentialing fee is $500 (normally $225 for other states).

KENTUCKY

	PTSponsor's Rating
Cost of Living	4
License Requirement	2
Salary Range	3
Overall	3

The Good: There is no limit in the number of times you can take the NPTE. This state also provides temporary license.

The Downside: Requirements include English proficiency exams, clinical internship (3-6 months), License from Country of Training and HIV-AIDS approved course.

The Bottom Line: The cost of living, license requirements and the salary are average.

Other Important Info: Clinical Internship: minimum 3 months with maximum 6 months; Temporary license is valid until the results of the 1st exam; complete an approved HIV/AIDS approved course.

LOUISIANA

	PTSponsor's Rating
Cost of Living	4
License Requirement	3
Salary Range	4
Overall	4

The Good: Louisiana offers a high salary for PTs. The cost of living is also low. There is no limit for the times you can take the NPTE.

The Downside: Clinical internship (with 1000 supervision hours) for 6 months is required. English proficiency exams are also part of the requirements.

The Bottom Line: Louisiana is an ideal place to work in, with the high salary, average requirements and low cost of living.

Other Important Info: Clinical Internship: 6 months with 1000 supervised clinical hours; Personal Interviews are conducted upon receipt of completed application and payment of fees. During the interview, a temporary permit may be issued.

MAINE

	PTSponsor's Rating
Cost of Living	2
License Requirement	1
Salary Range	3
Overall	2

The Good: Jurisprudence exams are not required.

The Downside: The cost of living is high, while the salary is relatively low. English proficiency exams are required. Temporary license is not issued to foreign-trained therapists. There is a 3-take limit to sit for the NPTE. There is a 6 month internship requirement.

The Bottom Line: This is not a good entry point for the foreign-trained physical therapist.

Other Important Info: Application fee consists of: Application-$75, License fee-$85, Criminal Background Fee-$15, Exam processing fee-$25. Clinical Internship: 6 Months; 3x permitted to sit for the NPTE then additional documentation will be required.

MARYLAND

	PTSponsor's Rating
Cost of Living	1
License Requirement	4

Salary Range	4
Overall	3

The Good: The salary for PTs here is one of the highest in the U.S. Clinical internship is also not required. Temporary licenses are issued to foreign PTs. There is also no limit to the number of times you can sit for NPTE.

The Downside: The cost of living is high in Maryland. English proficiency exams are required.

The Bottom Line: Aside from the high cost of living, Maryland is a good entry point for foreign physical therapists. They provide temporary license and there is no clinical internship requirement.

Other Important Info: Temporary license valid for 90 days; Jurisprudence exam passing score is 90%. All applicants must have a social security number.

MASSACHUSETTS

	PTSponsor's Rating
Cost of Living	2
License Requirement	2
Salary Range	4
Overall	3

The Good: There is no limit to the number of times you can sit for the exam. Clinical internship is not required.

The Downside: TOEFL is required. They do not provide a temporary license. Licensure in Country of Training is required.

The Bottom Line: This is an average state. The salary, cost of living and license requirement are all average.

MICHIGAN

	PTSponsor's Rating
Cost of Living	3
License Requirement	3
Salary Range	4
Overall	3

The Good: The salary range in Michigan is one of the highest in the U.S. The cost of living is average. They do not require clinical internship and license from country of training. There is also no limit in taking the NPTE.

The Downside: English proficiency exams are part of the requirements. They do not issue temporary licenses.

The Bottom Line: This is an ideal state to practice physical therapy for foreign trained physical therapists.

Other Important Info: Application is valid for 2 years only.

MINNESOTA

	PTSponsor's Rating
Cost of Living	3
License Requirement	3
Salary Range	3
Overall	3

The Good: They issue temporary licenses to foreign PTs, which they refer to as supervised traineeship. You can sit for NPTE for as many times as needed.

The Downside: Clinical internship (6 months, for 40 hours/week) and English proficiency exams are required.

The Bottom Line: Minnesota has average requirements and cost of living, however, the salary for physical therapists is low.

Other Important Info:

Clinical Internship: 6 months (40 hours per week); Application fee is $150= Permanent licensure fee (100) + Exam fee (50); completion of malpractice history form is required.

MISSISSIPPI

	PTSponsor's Rating
Cost of Living	5
License Requirement	2
Salary Range	4
Overall	4

The Good: If you haven't availed of a Social Security Number yet, you can show your copy of H1B Visa, INS Form I-94 to prove that your stay in the U.S. is valid. They give temporary license to those who have a current license in a jurisdiction which has a higher requirement than Mississippi.

The Downside: You are only allowed 5 attempts for the NPTE. Also, English proficiency exams are required.

The Bottom Line: The salary and cost of living are both low. The license requirements are just average.

Other Important Info: 5x permitted to sit for the exam regardless if taken in any other jurisdiction, after failing 2x, you are required to take remedial coursework.

MISSOURI

	PTSponsor's Rating
Cost of Living	5
License Requirement	3
Salary Range	3
Overall	4

The Good: Living in Missouri is cheap. They do not require clinical internship. If you don't have a Social Security number yet, you can furnish a copy of your visa or passport identification number in your application.

The Downside: You can take the NPTE up to three (3) times only. English proficiency exams are also required.

The Bottom Line: Both the cost of living and salary are low.

Other Important Info: 3x permitted to sit for the exam; Without SSN, you can present a copy of your visa or passport identification number.

MONTANA

	PTSponsor's Rating
Cost of Living	3
License Requirement	3
Salary Range	2
Overall	3

The Good: Clinical internship is not required in Montana. They also issue temporary licenses to foreign-trained physical therapists.

The Downside: The salary is low. They require English proficiency exams. You are only allowed 4 attempts on the NPTE.

The Bottom Line: License requirement and the cost of living are average. The catch is the low salary. After failing the NPTE 3x, remedial coursework is required. Application process may take 120 days.

NEBRASKA

	PTSponsor's Rating
Cost of Living	5
License Requirement	4

Salary Range	3	
Overall	4	

The Good: The cost of living is low. Clinical internship is not a requirement. There is no limit in the number of times you can take the NPTE. They also provide temporary licenses.

The Downside: Jurisprudence and English proficiency exams are required.

The Bottom Line: The cost of living is low; the salary range is average and not a lot of requirements from the state. It is a good state to start for a foreign-trained physical therapist.

Other Important Info: Temporary license valid until results of 1st exam; application fee is a range $26-52; jurisprudence exam is $50.00. Sitting fee for jurisprudence is $25.

NEVADA

	Therapists' Rating	PTSponsor's Rating
Cost of Living	2	2
License Requirement	0	0
Salary Range	5	5
Overall	2	2

The Good: Nevada offers one of the highest salary ranges in the U.S.

The Downside: There are lots of requirements-- English proficiency exams, clinical internship and license from country of training.

The Bottom Line: The cost of living here is high, but is evened out by the high salary. However, this is not a good entry point for a foreign physical therapist because of the numerous requirements.

Other Important Info: Clinical Internship: equal to an accredited program; after failing the NPTE 2x remedial coursework is required; fingerprinting fee is $45, application process takes 4-5 weeks.

Foreign PTs' Comment:" I had difficulty applying to this state because you have to be licensed in your own country. However, I like this state. The lights and shows are very remarkable."- M. R.

NEW HAMPSHIRE

PTSponsor's Rating

Cost of Living	1
License Requirement	2
Salary Range	3
Overall	2

The Good: No jurisprudence exam, no clinical internship.

The Downside: Salary is relatively low. Cost of living is relatively high. They do not provide temporary licenses to foreign physical therapists.

The Bottom Line:

This state has high cost of living, low salary and a long list of license requirements. It is not a good entry point.

Other Important Info:

No limit on the number of times you are allowed to sit for the NPTE, however, after failing 4-5x, you are required to take remedial coursework.

NEW JERSEY

	Therapists' Rating	PTSponsor's Rating
Cost of Living	1	1
License Requirement	0	2
Salary Range	5	4

The Ultimate Guide to Foreign-Trained Physical Therapists Wishing to Work in the US

Overall	2	2

The Good: New Jersey has one of the highest salary for physical therapists in the U.S. There is no limit on the number of times you can take the NPTE.

The Downside: Despite the high salary, the cost of living is also high. English proficiency exams are also required.

The Bottom Line: If you can cope with the list of requirements and the high cost of living, the high salary makes it worthwhile.

NEW MEXICO

	PTSponsor's Rating
Cost of Living	3
License Requirement	3
Salary Range	3
Overall	3

The Good: They do not require English proficiency exams and clinical internship. They also issue temporary licenses to foreign physical therapists.

The Downside: The low salary and the five-time limit to sit for NPTE are something to be considered. Remedial coursework is required after 2 failed attempts.

The Bottom Line: What makes this place a good state to practice is the average cost of living and the issuance of a temporary license. You don't have to go through clinical internship and if you have passed your local board exams for physical therapy, you won't find it hard to land a job here.

Other Important Info: Temporary license is valid for six months with renewal for six months for justifiable cause; No limit to sit for the NPTE, however, after failing 2x, you are required to take remedial coursework.

NEW YORK

	Therapists' Rating	PTSponsor's Rating
Cost of Living	1	1
License Requirement	5	5
Salary Range	4	4
Overall	3	3

The Good: New York is an ideal entry point for a foreign physical therapist. Clinical internship and TOEFL are not required. There is no limit in the number of times you are allowed to take the NPTE. They also issue temporary licenses.

The Downside: The cost of living is high, while the salary is just average.

The Bottom Line: Because of few requirements and average salary, this state is a good place to start.

Other Important Info: Credentialing: NYS Verification is different from the standard FCCPT credentialing; credentialing can also be completed by CGFNS credentials verification process; Temporary license is valid for 6 months.

NORTH CAROLINA

	PTSponsor's Rating
Cost of Living	4
License Requirement	2
Salary Range	4
Overall	3

The Good: Living in North Carolina is quite cheap. And they do not require clinical internship.

The Downside: There are many licensure requirements which include English proficiency exams and remedial coursework after failing the NPTE twice.

The Bottom Line: This state is average. The numerous licensure requirements could be worth accomplishing because of the state's low cost of living and high salary.

Other Important Info:

120 semester hours required-- 60 professional, 42 general ed, 21 can be taken as CLEP before 2003. After 2003, education must be equivalent to CAPTE approved PT program (post baccalaureate degree).

NORTH DAKOTA

	PTSponsor's Rating
Cost of Living	4
License Requirement	1
Salary Range	3
Overall	3

The Good: The cost of living in N. Dakota is low.

The Downside: There are many requirements such as English proficiency exams and clinical internship. Remedial coursework is also required after 2 failed attempts on the NPTE. The salary is low.

The Bottom Line: Because of the many requirements and low salary, this is not an ideal state for foreign trained physical therapists.Clinical Internship: 6 months; No limit to sit for the NPTE, however, after failing 2x, you are required to take remedial coursework.

OHIO

	Therapists' Rating	PTSponsor's Rating
Cost of Living	4	4
License Requirement	1	2
Salary Range	5	4
Overall	3	3

The Good: The salary range is high, while the cost of living is relatively low. There is no limit to the number of times you can sit for NPTE. The state does not require clinical internship.

The Downside: They require English proficiency exams and license from country of training. They do not issue temporary licenses.

The Bottom Line: The median annual wage in Ohio ranks 9th among the highest and the cost of living is low.

Other Important Info: No limit to sit for the NPTE, however, after failing 3x, you are required to take remedial coursework. Visa screen is required (can be obtained from FCCPT/ CGFNS); Required general education courses: humanities, 2 courses each of chemistry and physics with lab; biological sciences, social sciences, behavioral sciences and mathematics.

OKLAHOMA

	PTSponsor's Rating
Cost of Living	5
License Requirement	1
Salary Range	3
Overall	3

The Good: Oklahoma has one of the lowest cost of living in the U.S. The salary is relatively high. Foreign physical therapists are also issued temporary licenses.

The Downside: Passing your local board exams and English proficiency exams are part of the license requirements. You have three months to complete 800 hours of clinical internship. The limit for taking the NPTE is three times only.

The Bottom Line: The license requirements are many. The high salary and low cost of living, however, makes it worthwhile.

Other Important Info: Temporary license is valid until the next board meeting (may be extended). 3x allowed to sit for exam; after 2nd failure, must have study plan approved by Committee; licensure in country of training is required, clinical internship is 800 hours to be completed at a minimum of 120 days; 3 letters of recommendation required.

OREGON

	PTSponsor's Rating
Cost of Living	2
License Requirement	2
Salary Range	3
Overall	2

The Good: Clinical internship is not required, and the salary is relatively high.

The Downside: English proficiency and jurisprudence exams are required. Social Security number is also a requirement. You have to take a remedial coursework after failing the NPTE for the third time , and you can only take the NPTE for up to five times. The cost of living is high.

The Bottom Line: Despite the fact that the state offers a relatively high salary, you have to consider the high cost of living and the long list of licensure requirements.

Other Important Info: 5x limit to sit for the NPTE, however, after failing 3x, you are required to take remedial coursework; social security is required, 120 semester hours required, general education 54, professional education 69. See website for specific subjects required.

PENNSYLVANIA

	Therapists' Rating	PTSponsor's Rating
Cost of Living	2	2
License Requirement	1	1
Salary Range	4	4
Overall	2	2

The Good: English proficiency exams are not included in the list of licensure requirements.

The Downside: Living here is quite expensive. Among the requirements is a **12** month clinical internship and you can only take the NPTE twice.

The Bottom Line: The salary and cost of living here is high. There is also a long list of requirements before you can get a license.

Other Important Info: Clinical Internship: 12 months; After failing the NPTE 2x, you are required to take remedial coursework.

Foreign PTs' Comment: "PA only accepts license by endorsement for foreign trained PTs. SSN is required"- R. R.

RHODE ISLAND

	PTSponsor's Rating
Cost of Living	1
License Requirement	2
Salary Range	5
Overall	3

The Good: Clinical internship and English proficiency exams are not required.

The Downside: The cost of living in Rhode Island is high. If you failed the NPTE for three times, you have to take remedial coursework.

The Bottom Line: License requirements are quite numerous. The cost of living is high, while the salary range is just average.

Other Important Info: No limit to sit for the NPTE, however, after failing 3x, you are required to take remedial coursework; license application is valid for 1 year only; license processing is 4-6 weeks.

SOUTH CAROLINA

PTSponsor's Rating

Cost of Living	4
License Requirement	1
Salary Range	4
Overall	3

The Good: The salary is high and the cost of living is low.

The Downside: This state requires English proficiency exams and 1000 clinical internship hours. They also do not provide temporary license. You can only take the NPTE for up to three times.

The Bottom Line: The cost of living and salary are alright, but when it comes to licensure, they have many requirements.

Other Important Info: Clinical Internship: 1000 clinical hours; 3x limit to sit for the NPTE, however, after failing 2x, you are required to take remedial coursework.

SOUTH DAKOTA

PTSponsor's Rating

Cost of Living	5
License Requirement	3
Salary Range	3
Overall	4

The Good: Clinical internship is not included in the licensure requirements. There is no limit to the number of times you can take the NPTE. South Dakota has one of the lowest costs of living in the U.S.

The Downside: The salary range here is relatively low. English proficiency exams are part of the requirements. They do not issue temporary license to foreign trained physical therapists.

The Bottom Line: The cost of living and salary are low. Requirements are just average. This is not a bad entry point for a foreign physical therapist.

TENNESSEE

	PTSponsor's Rating
Cost of Living	5
License Requirement	1
Salary Range	4
Overall	3

The Good: The salary is high while the cost of living is low.

The Downside: TOEFL and 480 hour of clinical internship are part of the requirements. You have to take remedial coursework after failing the NPTE twice.

The Bottom Line: This is a state where cost of living and salary are very good. However, Tennessee has one of the most extensive list of license requirements. 480 hours of clinical internship shall be accomplished at a rate of no more than 40 hours or no less than 20 hours per week; No limit to sit for the NPTE, however, after failing 2x, you are required to take remedial coursework; application on file for 1 year only.

TEXAS

	Therapists' Rating	PTSponsor's Rating
Cost of Living	5	5
License Requirement	1	2
Salary Range	5	5
Overall	3.5	4

The Good: Texas is on the top 5 states which offer the highest salary. It also ranks 2nd on the states with a low cost of living. They also provide temporary license to foreign physical therapists.

The Downside: You have to pass your local physical therapy board exams. You have to acquire 60 general education credits, 72 professional education credits and at least 23 hours of clinical internship. This state is not very foreign-trained therapist friendly.

The Bottom Line: It is hard to get into this state for someone with a bachelor's degree.

Other Important Info: Also accepts Robert Watkins at UT Austin for credentialing; Temporary license valid until results of first exam; 8x limit to sit for the NPTE, however, after failing 2x, you are required to take remedial coursework; Board sends visa letter upon request, 60 general education credits, 72 professional education (90 after 2008), 15-23 clinical education; licensure in country of training is required.

Foreign PTs' Comments: "This state has very low cost of living, and very high salary. However, Texas is hard to apply to. It's like an entirely different country; it has different rules and standards, mostly higher that other states."- E.C

"Bad: The board accepts up to 12 credits through CLEP. That's a big drawback."- N. N.

UTAH

	PTSponsor's Rating
Cost of Living	3
License Requirement	4
Salary Range	3
Overall	3

The Good: English proficiency exams and clinical internship are not required. There is no limit in the number of times you can take the NPTE.

The Downside: The state does not provide temporary license to foreign-trained physical therapists. The salary range is low.

The Bottom Line: The state is average.

Other Important Info: If social security number is not provided, the application is incomplete and may be denied.

VERMONT

	PTSponsor's Rating
Cost of Living	1
License Requirement	5
Salary Range	3
Overall	3

The Good: Vermont has few license requirements. They do not require English proficiency exams and clinical internship. There is no NPTE limit. They also issue temporary licenses for foreign physical therapists.

The Downside: The cost of living is high while the salary is low.

The Bottom Line: Although license requirements here are few, the salary is relatively low and the cost of living is high.

VIRGINIA

	PTSponsor's Rating
Cost of Living	2
License Requirement	2
Salary Range	4
Overall	3

The Good: Virginia provides high salaries for physical therapists. Foreign physical therapists are also issued with a temporary license.

The Downside: English proficiency exams and 1000 clinical internship hours are part of the licensure requirements.

The Bottom Line: The salary is high, and the cost of living in Virginia is high too. They have a long list of requirements. Clinical Internship: 1000 hours; Temporary license valid for 90 days; no limit to sit for the NPTE, however, after failing 3x, you are required to take remedial coursework; application will be kept on file for 1 year only.

WASHINGTON

	Therapists' Rating	PTSponsor's Rating
Cost of Living	2	2
License Requirement	2	2
Salary Range	2	4
Overall	2	3

The Good: Salary is high. Clinical internship is not required in order to get a license.

The Downside: AIDS Education, jurisprudence and English proficiency exams are required. The cost of living in Washington is high. Foreign physical therapists are not issued a temporary license. After failing the NPTE for the second time, you have to take a remedial coursework.

The Bottom Line: The salary and cost of living are high. Licensure requirements are many. You need to have 50 general education credits, 69 professional credits. This is not an ideal state for a foreign physical therapist with a bachelor's degree.

Other Important Info: 4x limit to sit for the NPTE, however, after failing 2x, you are required to take remedial coursework; application process 2-3 months, AIDS Education required; 50 gen ed credits, 69 prof ed credits.

WEST VIRGINIA

	PTSponsor's Rating
Cost of Living	3
License Requirement	3
Salary Range	4
Overall	3

The Good: West Virginia offers a relatively high salary. Foreign physical therapists are provided a temporary license. There is no limit to take NPTE.

The Downside: English proficiency exams and 800-hour clinical internship are required.

The Bottom Line: The salary is high, while the cost of living and license requirements are average.

Other Important Info: Clinical Internship: 800 hours; Temporary license valid until results of 1st exam; licensing process takes 4-6 weeks.

WISCONSIN

	PTSponsor's Rating
Cost of Living	4
License Requirement	4
Salary Range	4
Overall	4

The Good: Clinical internship is not required. They also issue temporary licenses to foreign trained physical therapists.

The Downside: Jurisprudence and English proficiency exams are required.

The Bottom Line: The salary is high, and the cost of living is low. The license requirements are quite few.

Other Important Info:

Temporary license fee is $10.00, Jurisprudence Exam is $57.00

WYOMING

	PTSponsor's Rating
Cost of Living	3
License Requirement	2
Salary Range	3
Overall	3

The Good: Clinical internship is not required.

The Downside: English proficiency exams are required, and temporary license is not available for foreign physical therapists. There is a two-take limit to sit for the NPTE.

The Bottom Line: Both salary and cost of living are average. The requirements are quite many.

Other Important Info:

2x limit to sit for the NPTE; application is valid for 1 year only. (States, n.d.)

This list is provided to you through the reviews from our website. If you notice any errors, please contact us through our website. You are also free to add reviews on our website.

State	Address	Phone	Fax	Email
Alabama	Alabama Board of Physical Therapy 100 N Union Street Suite 724 Montgomery, AL 36130-5040	(334) 242-4064	(334) 242-3288	N K . H o r n e r @ pt.alabama.gov
Alaska	State PT & OT Board Dept. of Community & Economic Dev.333 Willoughby Avenue, 9th FloorJuneau, AK 99811	(907) 465-3262	(907) 465-2974	J u d y _ W e s k e @ commerce.state. ak.us
Arizona	Arizona State Board of Physical Therapy 4205 North 7th Avenue Suite 208 Phoenix, AZ 85013	(602) 274-0236	(602) 274-1378	h e i d i . h e r b s t - p a a k k o n e n @ ptboard.state.az.us
Arkansas	Arkansas State Board of Physical Therapy 9 Shackleford Plaza Suite 3 Little Rock, AR 72211	(501) 228-7100	(501) 228-0294	arptb@sbcglobal. net
California	Physical Therapy Board of California 1418 Howe Avenue Suite 16 Sacramento, CA 95825	(916) 561-8200	(916) 263-2560	pt@dca.ca.gov
Colorado	Colorado Physical Therapy Licensure Division of Registrations 1560 Broadway, Suite 1340 Denver, CO 80202-5146	(303) 894-7851	(303) 894-7693	pt@dora.state.co.us

The Ultimate Guide to Foreign-Trained Physical Therapists Wishing to Work in the US

State	Address	Phone	Fax	Email
Connecticut	Office of Practitioner Licensing and Certification 410 Capitol Ave.,MS#12APP Hartford, CT 06134-0308	(860) 509-8377	(860) 509-8457	oplc.dph@po.state.ct.us
Delaware	Division of Professional Regulation 861 Silver Lake Blvd., Ste #203 Cannon Bldg Dover, DE 19904-2467	(302) 744-4500	(302) 739-2711	sandra.wagner@state.de.us
District of Columbia	D.C. Board of Physical Therapy Health Professional Licensing Administration 717 14th Street, NW, Suite 600 Washington, DC 20005	(202) 724-8739	(202) 727-8471	gabrielle.schultz@dc.gov
Florida	MQA/Board of Physical Therapy Practice Bin C-05 4052 Bald Cypress Way Tallahassee, FL 32399-3255	(850) 245-4373	(850) 414-6860	health@doh.state.fl.us
Georgia	Georgia Board of Physical Therapy 237 Coliseum Drive Macon, GA 31217-3858	(478) 207-2440	(478) 207-1434	dwalker@sos.state.ga.us
Hawaii	Hawaii Dept. of Commerce & Consumer Affairs PO Box 3469 Honolulu, HI 96801	(808) 586-2694	(808) 586-2874	phys_therapy@dcca.hawaii.gov

State	Address	Phone	Fax	Email
Idaho	Bureau of Occupational Licenses, Owyhee Plaza 1109 Main St. Suite 220 Boise, ID 83702	(208) 334-3233	(208) 334-3945	ibol@ibol.idaho.gov
Illinois	Department of Professional Regulation Attn: Health Services Section 320 W. Washington St., 3rd Floor Springfield, IL 62786	(217) 782-8556	none	none
Indiana	Indiana Physical Therapy Committee 402 West Washington Street Room W072 Indianapolis, IN 46204	(317) 234-2051	(317) 233-4236	pla6@pla.in.gov
Iowa	Iowan Dept of Public Health Lucas State Office Bldg. 321 E 12th Street, 5th Floor Des Moines, IA 50319-0075	(515) 281-4413	(515) 281-3121	jmanning@idph.state.ia.us
Kansas	Kansas State Board of Healing Arts Physical Therapy Examining Committee 235 S. Topeka Blvd. Topeka, KS 66614	(785) 296-8563	(785) 296-0852	Klenahan@ksbha.ks.gov

The Ultimate Guide to Foreign-Trained Physical Therapists Wishing to Work in the US

State	Address	Phone	Fax	Email
Kentucky	Kentucky Board of Physical Therapy 312 Whittington Parkway Suite 102 Louisville, KY 40222	(502) 429-7140	(502) 429-7142	becky.klusch@ ky.gov
Louisiana	State Board of PT Examiners 104 Fairlane Dr. Lafayette, LA 70507	(337) 262-1043	(337) 262-1054	lsbpte@laptboard. org
Maine	Maine Department of Professional and Financial Regulation Office of Licensing and Registration 35 State House Station Augusta, ME 04333-0035	(207) 624-8603	(207) 624-8637	kelly.l.mclaughlin@ maine.gov
Maryland	Brd of Physical Therapy Examiners 4201 Patterson Ave., #223 Baltimore, MD 21215-2299	(410) 764-4752	(410) 358-1183	tyminska@dhmh. state.md.us
Massachusetts	Brd of Allied Health Professionals Division of Registration 239 Causeway St., Ste 500 Boston, MA 02114	(617) 727-9964	(617) 727-2669	ann.constable@ state.ma.us
Michigan	611 West Ottawa 1st Floor Lansing, MI 48909-7518	(517)335-0918	(517) 373-2179	bhphelp@michigan. gov

State	Address	Phone	Fax	Email
Minnesota	Minnesota Board of Physical Therapy 2829 University Ave., SE Ste 420 Minneapolis, MN 55414-3245	(612) 627-5406	(612) 627-5403	stephanie.lunning@ state.mn.us
Mississippi	Mississippi State Board of PT PO Box 55707 Jackson, MS 39296-5707	(601) 939-5124	(601) 939-5246	info@msbpt.state. ms.us
Missouri	Advisory Commision for Professional PTs and PTAs P.O. Box 4 Jefferson, MO 65102	(573) 751-0098	(573) 751-3166	healingarts@pr.mo. gov
Montana	Board of Physical Therapy 301 S. Park, 4th Floor P.O. Box 200513 Helena, MT 59620	(406) 841-2395	(406) 841-2305	dlibsdptp@mt.gov
Nebraska	Board of Physical Therapy Division of Public Health, Licensure Unit 301 Centennial Mall, PO Box 94986 Lincoln, NE 68509-4986	(402) 471-2299	(402)471-3577	irene.eckman@ dhhs.ne.gov
Nevada	NV State Bd of Physical Therapy Examiners 810 S. Durango Dr. Suite 109 Las Vegas, NV 89145	(702) 876-5535	(702)876-2097	atresca@govmail. state.nv.us

The Ultimate Guide to Foreign-Trained Physical Therapists Wishing to Work in the US

State	Address	Phone	Fax	Email
New Hampshire	PT Governing Brd. of N.Hampshire Ofc. of Allied Health Professionals 2 Industrial Park Dr. Concord, NH 03301	(603) 271-8389	(603) 271-6702	tina.kelley@nh.gov
New Jersey	New Jersey State Board of PT PO Box 45014	Newark, NJ 07101	none	http://www.state.nj.us/lps/ca/medical/pt.htm
New Mexico	NM Physical Therapy Board PO Box 25101 Sante Fe, NM 87505	(505) 476-4880	(505) 476-4645	physicaltherapy@state.nm.us
New York	Office of the Professions NYS Education Dept 89 Washington Ave. Albany, NY 12234	(518) 474-3817 x180	(518) 402-5944	PTBD@mail.nysed.gov
North Carolina	N.Carolina Board of Physical Therapy 18 W. Colony Pl., #140 Durham, NC 27705	(919) 490-6393	919-490-5106	bfmassey@mindspring.com
North Dakota	State Examining Committee for PT PO Box 69 Grafton, ND 58237	(701) 352-0125	(701) 352-3093	ndptboard@gra.midco.net
Ohio	Ohio Occupational Therapy, PT & Athletic Trainers Board 77 South High Street., 16th Fl. Columbus, OH 43215-6108	(614) 466-3774	(614) 995-0816	board@otptat.ohio.gov

State	Address	Phone	Fax	Email
Oklahoma	Board of Medical Licensure & Supervision Physical Therapy Advisory Committee 5104 N. Francis, Suite C Oklahoma, OK 73118-0256	(405)848-6841	(405) 848-8240	kplant@osbmls.state.ok.us
Oregon	Oregon Physical Therapy Licensing Board 800 NE Oregon St., Suite 407 Portland, OR 97232-2187	(971) 673-0200	(971) 673-0226	physical.therapy@state.or.us
Pennsylvania	Pennsylvania State Brd of Physical Therapy P.O. Box 2649 Harrisburg, PA 17105-2649	(717) 783-7134	(717) 787-7769	st-physical@state.pa.us
Rhode Island	Rhode Island Dept. of Health 3 Capitol Hill, Room 104 Providence, RI 02908-5097	(401) 222-1750	(401)222-1272	maureen.slowik@health.ri.gov
South Carolina	South Carolina Board of Physical Therapy 110 Centerview Drive PO Box 11329 Columbia, SC 29211	(803) 896-4655	none	Reynoldsv@llr.sc.gov

State	Address	Phone	Fax	Email
South Dakota	SD State Board of Medical and Osteopathic Examiners 125 South Main Ave.Sioux Falls, SD 57104	(605) 367-7781	(605) 367-7786	sdbmoe@state.sd.us
Tennessee	Division of Health Related Boards Board of Occupational & PT 227 French Landing, Suite 300 Nashville, TN 37243	(615) 532-5132	(615) 532- 5164	Bonnie.Ferrell@state.tn.us
Texas	Texas Board of Physical Therapy Examiners 333 Guadalupe Suite 2-510 Austin, TX 78701-3942	(512) 305-6900	(512) 305-6951	info@ecptote.state.tx.us
Utah	Division of Occupational and Professional Licensing 160 E 300 South Box 146741 Salt Lake City, UT 84114	(801) 530-6621	(801) 530-6511	ntaxin@utah.gov
Vermont	Physical Therapy Advisors Office of Professional Regulation National Life Building, North, FL 2 Montpelier, VT 05620-3402	(802) 828-2191	(802) 828-2368	www.sec.state.vt.us
Virginia	Virginia Board of Physical Therapy Dept. of Health Professions 9960 Mayland Drive Suite 300 Richmond, VA 23233-1463	(804) 367-4630	none	Lisa.Hahn@dhp.virginia.gov

State	Address	Phone	Fax	Email
Washington	Washington Board of Physical Therapy PO Box 47867 Olympia, WA 98504-7867	(360) 236-4700	(360) 664-9077	https://fortress. wa.gov/doh/hpqal/ hps3/Physical_ Therapy/default. htm
West Virginia	WV Board of Physical Therapy 642 Davisson Run Road Clarksburg, WV 26301	none	none	wvbopt@yahoo.com
Wisconsin	WI Department of Regulation & Licensing 1400 E. Washington Ave., Room 178 PO Box 8935 Madison, WI 53708-8935	608.261.2378	(608) 267-3816	Thomas.Ryan@drl. state.wi.us
Wyoming	50 Wyoming Board of Physical Therapy 1800Carey Ave., 4th Floor Cheyenne, WY 82002	(307) 777-3507	(307) 777-3508	nbrown1@state. wy.us

The Ultimate Guide to Foreign-Trained Physical Therapists Wishing to Work in the US

Choosing a Sponsoring Employer

Things to Consider in Choosing an Employer to Sponsor You for a Visa

A sponsoring employer is one which legitimizes or pays for a program, project, visa, trip, or other initiative. In the case of foreign trained physical therapists, these employers sponsor for a visa. This will enable foreign trained physical therapists to work in the United States legally. Agencies provide health facilities with PT services, meaning they are the mediator between the foreign physical therapist and the healthcare facility.

1.   Type of Visa offered

For employment, an employer may sponsor you for a H1B or Green card. H1B will allow you to work faster (especially if the processing is expedited and you are lucky enough that the H1B quota is not yet reached.) This is valid for three years. This means that you also have to work for the same employer who sponsored you for that time.

On the other hand, a green card permits you to work in the US for ten years. You may also opt to be a U.S. citizen. It also requires you to work for only six months with your sponsor. You can work wherever you want after that. However, the process is long, taking one year or longer. If you can, having both can be very expedient.

Most employers will offer you H1b sponsorship. They will offer you a green card later, usually after six months. So, try to get a green card as soon as possible.

2.   Contract

Employers usually offer a contract of 2-3 years. If you can, get the shortest contract.

3.   Salary

The labor certification mandates the prevailing pay rate for each state. That is around $ 20-30 per hour. In a 40 hour work week, it would amount to an annual income of $

40,000- 50,000. Expect to get higher, but not too much. If you are a fresh graduate, asking $ 65,000 annually can be too much. Also consider the cost of living in a state. Even if a location is within the same state, the cost of living can be different.

4. Fees

Agencies earn by salary deduction. They will provide you with an estimate of hourly rate and charge the facility twice or thrice as much as your hourly rate. It is usually better to work for a direct employer.

5.   Benefits

After 4-6 months of employment, a two to three week vacation time (which could include or exclude holidays, personal days and sick leave), medical/dental insurance, tuition reimbursements and exam fee reimbursements are the ideal benefits. Agencies give at least 2 weeks of vacation time plus five holidays. Four or six months after your employment, you will be offered if you want medical insurance. Try to get as many benefits as you can.

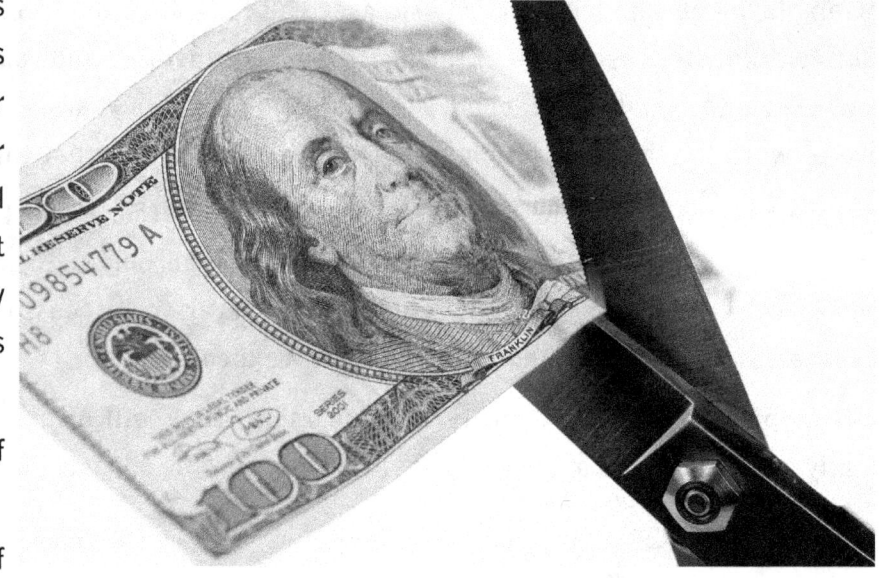

6.   Breach   of Contract

For   a   breach   of contract, agencies typically charge from $ 2,000 - $ 5,000. But there are contracts which will require you to pay over $ 50, 000. The $2,000-$ 5,000 charges as stated in the contract can be considered fair. So, have a lawyer to take care of this and explain the contract to you. This will prevent you from losing all your earnings if ever. There are also some contracts which are not valid. It all depends on the state's laws. If there is anything on the contract that seems vague to you, it is best to ask a lawyer to clarify it (Choosing an Agency to Sponsor you for a Visa, 2008).

The following is a list of some sponsoring agencies, along with their contact details, physical therapists review and reviews by the PTSponsor administration. The information provided here is just an assessment by PTSponsor's administration and physical therapists who have worked for these agencies. They just serve as hints of what it could be like to work for these agencies/companies and they are not necessarily a valid basis for judgment. It is your decision if you are going to try to work for these agencies.

RATINGS: (Scale of 1-5, with 5 being the highest)

BANNER HEALTH

Location: Works with Interstaff Manila

Phone: +1866-377-5627   Fax: not available

Website: www.bannerhealth.com   E-mail: not available

Therapists' Rating		PTSponsor Rating	
Annual Salary	3	Annual Salary	1
Length of Contract	5	Length of Contract	1
Benefits	5	Benefits	1
Breach of Contract	5	Breach of Contract	1
Overall	4.5	Overall	1

The Good: Banner Health gives out education assistance (scholarships and tuition reimbursement)

The Downside: Information about the agency is limited.

The Bottom Line: Interstaff Manila is their contact in the Philippines.

Testimonial:"I applied to them directly, not through Interstaff Manila. They are very reasonable and accommodating."-E. P.

ARDOR HEALTH SOLUTIONS

Location: 11555 Heron Bay Blvd, Suite 308 Coral Springs, FL 33076

Phone: +1866-425-5768   Fax: +1888-308-1147

Website: www.ardorhealth.com   E-mail: info@ardorhealth.com

Therapists' Rating		_PTSponsor's' Rating_	
Annual Salary	3	Annual Salary	1
Length of Contract	5	Length of Contract	3
Benefits	5	Benefits	5
Breach of Contract	5	Breach of Contract	1
Overall	4.5	Overall	3

The Good: Ardor Health Solutions give Free PPO Medical (CIGNA), Vision Care, Dental Insurance, and all paid Life Insurance. They also give Completion Bonuses (after every assignment), referral bonus plans, immediate travel reimbursements, private housing or housing allowance, CEU reimbursements and access to full time opportunities in the areas that you want to work in.

The Downside: There is no information provided about salary and breach of contract.

The Bottom Line: This agency would be a very good choice if you manage to get a good salary and breach of contract agreement.

Testimonial: "I have worked for them. They are reasonable. They have good benefits. A good company to work for." -C.C.

HORIZON HEALTH

Location: 2941 South Lake Vista Drive Lewisville, Texas 75067

Phone: 1-800-931-4646   Fax: 972.420.8252

Website: www.horizonhealth.com   Email: Mark.blakeney@horizonhealth.com

Therapists' Rating		PTSponsor's' Rating	
Annual Salary	4	Annual Salary	1
Length of Contract	4	Length of Contract	1
Benefits	5	Benefits	5
Breach of Contract	5	Breach of Contract	1
Overall	4.5	Overall	2

The Good: Offers many benefits such as Health Care Plan with medical, dental and pharmacy coverage; Group Life and Supplemental Life; Disability Insurance; Paid time off holidays, vacation days and sick days; 401 (k) Retirement Plan; Employee Assistance Program.

The Downside: Availability of information is limited.

The Bottom Line: Overall assessment is not possible due to lack of information.

Testimonial:

"I have worked for them and they give you all the benefits. Here in the United States, health insurance is very important. They provide this to you. They even pay you for holidays, sick days and vacation days. They also provide housing allowance. This amount will be calculated based on the amount of time you want to stay with them. There is no contract and therefore, no breach. I recommend them."   -M. L.

AXIOM LINK

Location: 60 Madison Ave, 8th floor New York, NY 10010

Phone: 1866-696-7991   Fax: 1-866-696-7991

Website: www.axiomlink.com   E-mail: jobs@axiomlink.com

Therapists' Rating		PTSponsor's Rating	
Annual Salary	5	Annual Salary	1
Length of Contract	3.5	Length of Contract	1
Benefits	4.5	Benefits	5
Breach of Contract	5	Breach of Contract	1
Overall	4	Overall	2

The Good: Up to $5,000 sign on bonus, comprehensive health insurance, dental, short term disability; 401k, paid time off, tuition and CEU assistance, relocation reimbursement.

The Downside: The agency only discusses matters regarding salary and contract with prospective employees, so be the one to contact them for more information.

The Bottom Line: Contact them for more information, if you find their offers reasonable.

Testimonial: "Great Company!! I have not yet taken a job with them yet but they are my number 1 pick."-M. A.

CROSS COUNTRY TRAVCORPS

Location: 6551 Park of Commerce Blvd. Boca Raton, FL 33487-8247

Phone: 1800-530-6125   Fax: not available

Website:www.crosscountryallied.com   E-mail: info@crosscountryallied.com

Therapists' Rating		*PTSponsor's Rating*	
Annual Salary	5	Annual Salary	5
Length of Contract	3.5	Length of Contract	3.5
Benefits	4.5	Benefits	4.5
Breach of Contract	5	Breach of Contract	5
Overall	4	Overall	4

The Good: Cross Country TravCorps gives $1000 referral bonus, free, private housing with amenities, health benefits, travel and license reimbursement.

The Downside: They offered information that length of contract is 18 months to 24 months. They said that longer contracts entail better housing benefits.

The Bottom Line: Not enough information is collected to make an accurate rating. It's up to you to contact them for more of your inquiries. If you want a permanent placement, you can try them.

RCM HEALTHCARE

Location: 575 8th Ave 6th floor New York, NY 10018

Phone: 212-221-1544   Fax: 212-869-4549

Website: http://www.rcmhealthcare.com   E-mail: healthcare@rcmt.com

Therapists' Rating		*PTSponsor's Rating*	
Annual Salary	4.5	Annual Salary	4
Length of Contract	2	Length of Contract	2
Benefits	5	Benefits	5
Breach of Contract	1	Breach of Contract	1
Overall	3	Overall	3

The Good: They offer these new salary rates for physical therapists: 1st year: $28.5, 2nd year: $29, 3rd year: $29.5 (Quoted at the time of writing.)

The Downside: They will offer you with a green card after two years of employment. A breach of contract can cost you $ 20,000 for legal fees which will be shouldered by you. You will be sued by this company if you breached your contract.

The Bottomline: Their services are only available in New Jersey, New York, Pennsylvania, Virginia and Maryland. If you can commit yourself to a three-year contract, this agency would be ideal to work for. If not, then you might want to avoid legal problems, choose another agency.

Testimonials:

"Thanks to RCM Health Care Services I was able to obtain a position with high pay and excellent benefits. My recruiter who worked with me was professional, dedicated and caring. I have worked with other staffing firms, but RCM is definitely number one. I would recommend RCM to anyone. Thank you again for finding me an incredible position and making my job search such a positive experience."-RCM Healthcare

"New salaries for PT's, 1st year 28.5, 2nd $29, 3rd $29.5. Medical, Dental, Vision, 401k, free life insurance, long term disability. free 2 months of housing, free flight, free immigration, free licenses. We work in NY, NJ, PA, MD, DC, and VA, not CT... You can bring your whole family. You are right about breach, we don't play games there, so people must be sure, that being said we have over 100 sponsored therapists currently working for us! Check out our video on our web site under foreign recruitment.www.rcmhealthcare. com. We have been in business for over 35 years now!"-E. M.

MEDICAL RESOURCES LLC

Location: 3155 West Big Beaver Rd. Suite 205 Troy, MI 48084

Phone: 1877-297-4084   Fax: +1248-649-4112

Website: not available   E-mail: ddelong@medical-resourcesllc.com

Therapists' Rating		PTSponsor's Rating	
Annual Salary	2	Annual Salary	1
Length of Contract	3	Length of Contract	1
Benefits	2	Benefits	3
Breach of Contract	3	Breach of Contract	1
Overall	2.5	Overall	2

The Good: Medical Resources LLC gives 401k, paid housing and travel allowance, medical benefits and malpractice insurance, $1000 sign on bonuses.

The Downside: Medical Resources LLC is a placement agency. The salary, contract length and breach will depend on the clinic or hospital where you will be assigned.

The Bottom Line: Since Medical Resources LLC is a placement agency, they cannot provide more information about the salary and contracts.

Testimonial: "They are a placement agency. It really depends where they place you. I got in a really busy clinic with few benefits. Some people have more luck than me."-J. S.

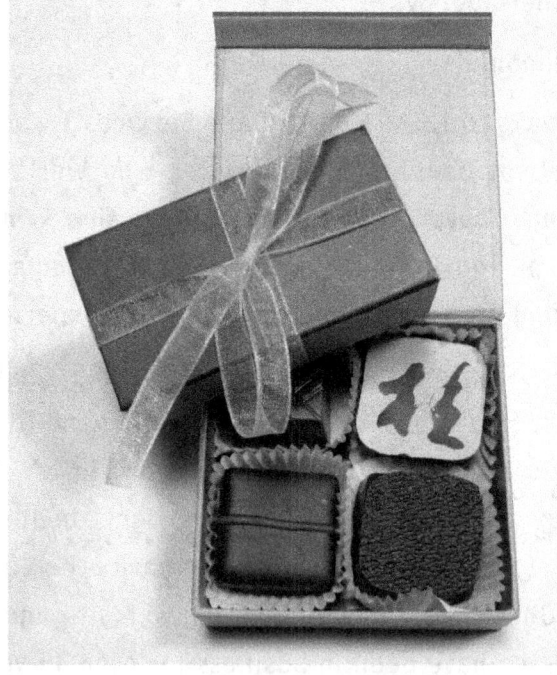

REHAB STAFFING, INC.

Location: 174 Grand St. White Plains, NY 10601

Phone:914 328-8077

Fax: not available

Website:www.rehabstaffinginc.com

Therapists' Rating		PTSponsor's Rating	
Annual Salary	3	Annual Salary	2
Length of Contract	2.5	Length of Contract	3
Benefits	3	Benefits	2
Breach of Contract	1	Breach of Contract	1
Overall	2	Overall	2

The Good: Rehab staffing provides 11 days vacation, 6 holidays, malpractice insurance and covers 50% of your health care insurance.

The Downside: A year after termination of contract, a non-compete clause should be provided.

The Bottom Line: Information about the breach of contract was not disclosed. However, the benefits and salary are quite good, thus, we give them a rating of 2.

Testimonials:"I have applied with them. Not a good choice."-Name withheld

"The contract is 2 years. Contract includes non-disclosure, non-solicitation, non-competition. You are responsible for licensing fees. They pay for professional liability insurance. 30 day notice required for resignation. Compensation is 35,000 until PT license is achieved then you will get 50,000. You get 11 personal/vacation/sick days each year. Holidays include New Year, Labor Day, Memorial Day, Independence Day, Thanksgiving and Xmas. Breach of contract is 10,000 dollars."-A. F.

"In this day and age, it's hard to find a company you can trust. With REHAB STAFFING, INC., the quality of service I received and continue to receive is outstanding. Keep up the good work!" – (from Rehab Staffing website)

"Thanks Janine, for allowing me to be part of this great organization. I love the company I am at and the people here are terrific !" – (from Rehab Staffing website)

"I have just signed another contract with you guys ! I've been here 5 years and it keeps on getting better." – (from Rehab Staffing website)

JUNO HEALTHCARE STAFFING

Location: 91-31 Queens Blvd, Suite 509 Elmhurst, NY 11373

Phone: 718-3967325   Fax: 718-3967328

Website: www.junohealthcare.com   E-mail: juno@junohealthcare.com

Therapists' Rating		PTSponsor's Rating	
Annual Salary	3	Annual Salary	3
Length of Contract	2	Length of Contract	2
Benefits	2	Benefits	3
Breach of Contract	1	Breach of Contract	1
Overall	2	Overall	2

The Good: Juno Healthcare Staffing sponsors physical therapists for an H1B visa.

The Downside: Contract is 3 years. We have been told that breach can go as high as 40,000.

The Bottom Line: If you plan to stay with this agency for 3 years, go ahead. Otherwise, be careful with your breach.

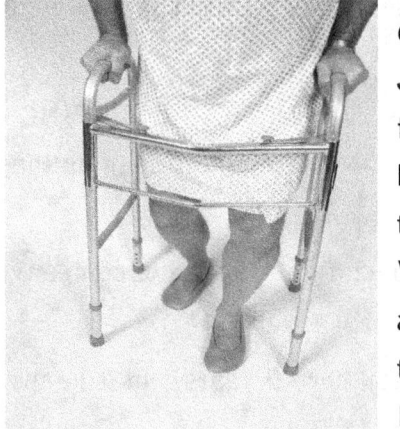

Testimonial: "You will pay JUNO the amount of $6,000.00 which will cover the following fees: USCIS filing fee, lawyer's professional fee, visa screen, administration fee, one-way airfare from the country of origin to the U.S. and initial housing accommodation. Contract is 3 years. In my contract, they said breach is: profits that JUNO would have earned had the Beneficiary not breached, amount spent by JUNO for the petition, actual damages including attorney's fees, litigation expenses and court fees. Salary is 25 per hour. Depending on how you work your deal, some I know get their CGFNS, TOEFL, TSE, Filing fee for immigration and Visa screen certificate fee reimbursed. Some also got free airfare, housing and accommodation assistance. Others got their reimbursement upon completion of the 3 year term."-R.R.

IRI REHAB STAFF

Location: 3910 Park Avenue Suite 3 Edison, NJ 08820

Phone: not available   Fax : not available

Website: www.irirehabstaff.com   E-mail: info@irirehabstaff.com

Therapists' Rating		PTSponsor's Rating	
Annual Salary	1	Annual Salary	3
Length of Contract	2	Length of Contract	3
Benefits	3	Benefits	5
Breach of Contract	2	Breach of Contract	1
Overall	2	Overall	3

The Good: IRI Rehab Staff gives $1500 reimbursement for exams and licensure, $1000 sign on bonus, free housing until you start working, airport pick-up, car loan if required, medical and dental benefits, 6 holidays, and 6 sick days; 10 vacation days, and overtime pay.

The Downside: Breach of contract costs up to $ 10,000, and hiring expenses.

The Bottom Line: Benefits and salary rate given by this company are competitive.

Testimonial:"If you need a sponsor, they will sponsor you. But they are not stellar or anything like that. They are average."-M. S.

MEDICAL SOLUTIONS PROVIDER LLC

Location: 2088, Route 130 N Monmouth Junction – 08852 NJ/Central

Phone: 732-398-1700   Fax: not available

Website: www.mspllc.com   E-mail: info@mspllc.com

Therapists' Rating		PTSponsor's Rating	
Annual Salary	1	Annual Salary	1
Length of Contract	3	Length of Contract	3
Benefits	3	Benefits	3
Breach of Contract	1	Breach of Contract	1
Overall	2	Overall	2

The Good: Contract is for 2 years. Medical Solutions Provider **LLC** gives medical insurance, along with 5 days paid time off, six holidays, liability insurance and a month of living accommodation.

The Downside: Salary is quite low, ranging from $ 40, 000-45,000 annually. The breach of contract is not clearly stated.

The Bottom Line: Try this agency with the risk of low salary and high breach of contract fines.

Testimonial: "2 year contract from the day you passed the exam. Rate is 20 per hour, at 40-hour workweek that is 41,600. If you fail the exam the second time, you will be terminated and will be returned to the country of origin upon the discretion of the employer. They provide one month free housing. They pay for 5 days sick/vacation/personal time, six paid holidays (New Year, Memorial Day, Independence Day, Labor Day, Thanksgiving, Christmas). They pay for the first year of your individual liability insurance. Breach of contract is 50% of said therapist's annual salary plus any additional expenses. You are not allowed to work for anyone within the 300 mile radius. Be careful, read their contract. I received 3 different contracts with 3 different wages and breaches!"-A.F.

AMERICAN MEDICAL MANAGEMENT OF NEW YORK

Location: 260 Middle Country Road, Bldy 3, Suite 9-A, Selden, New York 11784

Phone: +18774567799   Fax: not available

Website: not available   E-mail: not available

Therapists' Rating		_PTSponsor's Rating_	
Annual Salary	1	Annual Salary	2
Length of Contract	3	Length of Contract	3
Benefits	2	Benefits	2
Breach of Contract	1	Breach of Contract	1
Overall	1.5	Overall	2

The Good: The contract length is two years. The benefits include liability insurance, medical insurance, 1 week vacation and 6 holidays.

The Downside: You'll have to pay half of your annual salary for a breach of contract, which could be up to $ 20,000.

The Bottom Line: The benefits and the breach of contract are not very attractive.

Testimonial:

"I applied for this agency. They sent me the contract for me to sign. I did not sign it, it seems to me the contract is unfair."-J. W.

(Agencies, n.d.)

Preparing your Resume

An essential part of job seeking is distributing your resume. The resume is your passport to secure a job. This contains all the vital information that the employer needs to know about an applicant. This is decisive whether you will be hired or not. So what are the important things to remember when making your resume?

1.   List down all your information in a piece of paper

•   Contact details

•   Schools attended

•   Work experience

•   Seminars/workshops attended

•   Certificates

•   Special Skills/Abilities (related to job)

2.   Decide which format is most suitable for you. There are many types of formats, according to purpose and structure.

•   Functional

- Chronological

- Combination of the Two

- Targeted

3.   List down your probable character references. (Those people who the company/agency can contact for more information about you.)

The Resume Formats

Resumes can be categorized by their purpose and the presentation of vital information. Your qualifications will be judged on how you have presented your resume, although this is not the core basis for getting employed. But there are some things to remember in making an impressive resume. But before that, you have to know what kind of resume you have to make.

Functional

This type of resume highlights your skills, experience and accomplishments instead of your work history. This is recommended for someone who just made a career shift into physical therapy and for people who want to conceal gaps within their work history.

Example Outline:

John Doe
1234 Boulevard
Town, Province
(02) 123-4567
Email : email@email.com
OBJECTIVE
SUMMARY OF QUALIFICATIONS
PROFESSIONAL ACCOMPLISHMENTS
EDUCATION

Chronological

This type of resume prioritizes a record of your work history, starting from your most recent job to your first job. This is recommended for individuals who have more experiences.

Jane Doe
123 City, State
(02) 123-4567
Email : email@email.com
OBJECTIVE
WORK EXPERIENCE
EDUCATION

Targeted

A targeted resume presents skills relevant to the job that you are aspiring for. This kind of resume is customized to match the job description. This is also ideal if you had any other jobs aside from physical therapy, and that job can be irrelevant to health care and you want to omit it.

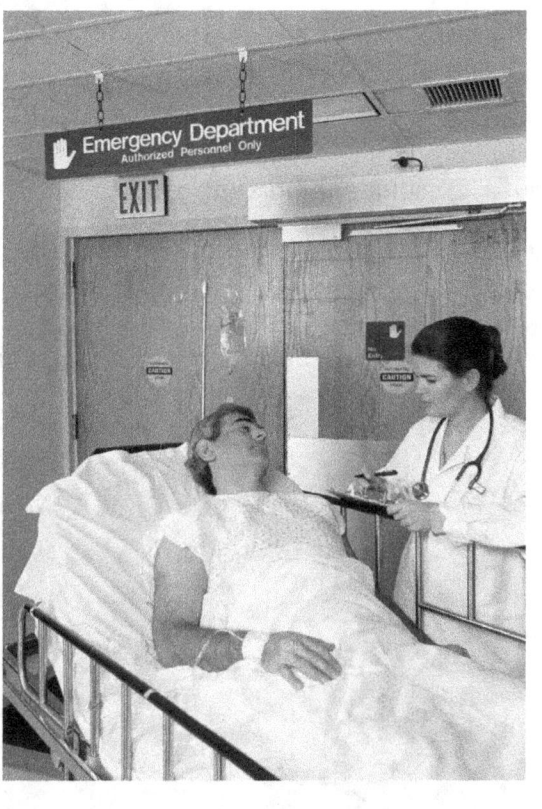

Combination of Functional and Chronological

A functional resume may highlight your skills, but it could leave the employer/agency in doubt about your qualifications if confirmation is concerned. On the other hand, a chronological resume may look so dull and boring. Getting the best of both worlds from these two resume formats can let you create a very good resume. It could be a functional combination, or a chronological combination. The functional format combination still has the tone of presenting your accomplishments and also lists work experience in the field of physical therapy, but it has the chronological format's list of relevant work experiences. The chronological combination format maintains setting down a job-by-job description, but also highlighting achievements and skills in physical therapy (Preparing a Resume, 2008).

Do's and Don'ts in Making a Resume

Your resume should be as brief as it can be. Having a very long resume can make the employer bored. Your resume should also state all the important information about you. So what are the things you have to remember while making your resume?

DO

• Include important contact details (telephone number, email)

• State your objective clearly. Avoid hesitant statements. Be direct to the point. Your objective answers the questions: What do I want to do? For whom? Where?

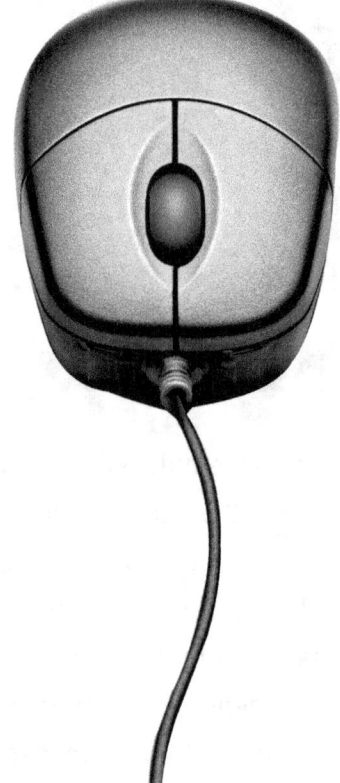

• Always check your spelling and grammar. Word processors can help detect obvious mistakes, but you should not solely rely on them. Have someone look at your resume and ask if they notice some mistakes.

• Make different versions of your resume. This could be extra work, but remember there is no such thing as a one-size-fits-all resume.

DON'T

...Lie. This is the most important rule in making your resume. Lying in your resume will bring you more trouble than you thought.

...Add references. Make it available upon request of the employer/agency.

...Add personal details such as religion, personal interests etc.

...State reasons for leaving/being terminated from a job. This could give bad impressions about you. Save it for the interview.

…Attach your photo. Some employers are inconsiderate enough to judge an applicant by their outer appearances. If they don't like you, they could disregard your qualifications and set you aside just because they don't like you. You want to present yourself during the interview. So if it is not required, don't attach your photo in your resume.

Permanent Placement Vs. Traveling

Definitions:

Permanent Placement: This generally means a job where you are placed for a definite period of time to last until the end of your contract. Typical assignment length is usually the length of the contract (1 year to 3 years).

Traveling: This indicates that a therapist will be transferred to different PT institutions/clinics/hospitals etc. This is done several times within a signed contract length. The length of each individual assignment depends on the agency, but commonly 13 weeks to 6 months assignments within a certain facility and a contract length of 1 to 3 years.

Requirements/Job Qualifications:

Permanent Placement: Any foreign-educated PT is qualified in this position as long as they have obtained a license within the state.

Traveling: This position usually calls for individuals who are single or married but without school aged children. This is not done to discriminate the individual, but to protect the PT from the possible family problems that may occur with constant moving. The job usually calls for individuals with 1 year driving experience and basic automotive maintenance skills.

Benefits:

Permanent Placement:

1.   Opportunity for career growth within the facility. Typically, agencies and direct hire facilities stipulate within contracts the length of time (usually one year) before requests for salary increase (and increase of managerial duties) can be made.

2.   Long-lasting professional relationships and friendships. Without the hassle of constant moving, you have the opportunity to make and foster long-lasting friendships. There is also the security in a workplace that cannot be achieved by traveling therapists.

Traveling:

1.   Free housing. Most, if not all traveling agencies offer free housing within the contract period. This is usually in the form of one bedroom apartment. This is great for those who have just migrated to the US because it cuts the costs. Usually, the traveling agency also pays for the furniture rental. Recruiters usually use this as a trump card because you can save a lot of money with free rent (you just have to pay for amenities). And they usually tell you that you can move in with literally only your suitcase. Appliances, bedsheets and curtains are provided by the agency.

2.   Free transportation or car loan plans. Newly migrated PTs have difficulty obtaining loans for cars; most agencies provide a company car or car loan plans that will be met throughout the contract period.

3.   Free gas: Most of the traveling PT's are given gas cards or reimbursed for job-related traveling.

4.   Free licensure processing. In endorsing your license, the agency will pay the fees for transfer to another state and help you obtain the license.

The Cons:

Permanent Placement:

1.   Usually there is no free housing. At most, there are units made available by the company at lower rates.

2.   Individuals who are unsatisfied with the work conditions of their current facility are stuck with them for the duration of the contract.

Traveling:

1.   Constant moving. Yes, traveling is great. But after a length of time, it becomes

boring. You may be assigned to a remote area. Recruiters constantly tell you that your preference in location will be given consideration in assignments, but at the end of the day, the agency will still place you in an area that would be most profitable for them.

2.   Families are the ones affected. It would be very difficult to remain a traveling physical therapist if your spouse is involved in a permanent placement position, PT related or not. Children also have a difficult time in adjusting to the constant change. As stated earlier, PTs with school age children are usually not given traveling jobs because it will affect the child's attendance in school (pisikal_terapist, 2008).

Some examples of agencies who offer permanent placement positions:

1.   Bilinguals Inc./Axiom Link: www.bilingualsinc.com

2.   O'Grady Peyton: www.ogradypeyton.com

Also offers traveling PT after finishing their contract or for US-grads

3.   Interface Rehab: www.interfacerehab.com

 Also offers traveling positions within CA

Note: CA is usually a difficult state to enter for migrating workers due to SSN requirements.

4.   Julie Edmunds Associates: http://www.juliaedmunds.com/

Some examples of agencies who offer traveling positions:

1.   Atlas Rehabilitation: www.atlasrehabilitation.com

2.   PPR Healthcare: www.pprhealthcare.com

(Permanent Placement vs. Travelling, 2008)

Choosing an Immigration Lawyer

When you plan to work in a foreign country, you have to get your immigration matters fixed first for a hassle free residence and career venture. This could be especially hard for someone who plans to work in a foreign country for the first time. Each country has its different immigration laws. Where do you find help about these immigration law matters, and also some more help when it comes to dealing with your employer? It would be best to get yourself an immigration lawyer. Immigration lawyers will explain to you these immigration laws, and also translate immigration law and policy for you to understand these things better. They will be the one to interpret these laws for you. They can help you hasten your visa application process, or let them take a look at your contract (with your employer) to be sure that what is stated in your contract is fair or not. They can also help you sue abusive agencies or companies you have worked for. PTSponsor has listed some immigration law firms along with reviews and ratings given by PTSponsor users and administration.

AMES IMMIGRATION

472 South Salina Street, Suite 501 Syracuse, NY 13202

Phone: 315-423-0282   Fax: 315-476-9466

Website: www.amesimmigrationlaw.com   E-mail: info@amesimmigrationlaw.com

Therapists' Ratings		PTSponsor's Rating	
Fees	5	Fees	4
Speed	5	Speed	5
Accessibility	5	Accessibility	5
Overall	5	Overall	5

The Good: They are very friendly. They quickly respond to their client's needs.

The Downside: They charge more than $ 3, 500 worth of legal fees for H1B, and more than $ 5,000 for a green card.

The Bottom Line: if you need fast and reliable legal assistance, their services are worth a try, however, you must be ready to spend a lot of money.

Testimonial: "I was quoted the same rates. I think that is too much money. Almost 10,000 dollars to get a green card!"- R. D.

CATHERINE MAY CO & Associates

10 5th St., Suite 103, Valley Stream NY 11581

Phone: 516-284-7445   Fax: 718-412-3212

Website: usaimmigration101.com   E-mail: cco@NyLegalOption.com

Therapists' Rating		PTSponsor's Rating	
Fees	4	Fees	3
Speed	5	Speed	5
Accessibility	5	Accessibility	5
Overall	4.5	Overall	4

The Good: They are very fast and easy to talk with.

(Information from their website): Catherine May Co & Associates is a firm of experienced U.S. immigration lawyers dedicated to serving individuals and businesses through the practice of immigration law. We handle immigration matters for clients throughout the United States and the world in an expeditious and personalized manner. Our mission is to provide you with individual attention and professional service at every step on the path toward achieving your immigration goals.

U.S. immigration law is extremely complex and only a professional can assist you through the process. Our immigration attorneys provide immediate attention to our clients to ensure that every petition is diligently prepared and thoroughly analyzed. For individuals, we provide assistance with work visas, family petitions, marriage and fiancé visas, investor visas, asylum, deportation defense and citizenship. For businesses, our pledge is to provide strategic, personalized guidance tailored to achieve your goals in establishing a U.S. affiliate or subsidiary, transferring employees to the U.S. or investing in the U.S. We recognize the immigration process is full of challenges, obstacles, and unforeseen hazards. Thus, we work diligently to help our clients achieve their immigration objective.

Our Firm stays up-to-date with rapidly changing laws and growing customer expectations. Our staff utilizes advanced office technology for document creation, client case management, communication, and internal coordination. We carefully and capably manage client case work - from brief, simple processes to complex, long-term cases. Our firm strives to maintain a superior quality of work and full attention to detail. We believe that the satisfaction of each of our clients is paramount.

The Downside: Their fees are on the high side.

The Bottom Line: If you want a lawyer who will take care of your legal needs and if you want speed and efficiency, you might consider getting a lawyer from this firm.

Testimonial: "I have contract with an employer. They treated me so poorly, I resigned. This law firm defended me."- R.R.

"Received my green card via EB2 in 3 months!!! I am really happy and could not thank this office more!" G.T.

"I was a victim of a immigration scam and the USCIS found me guilty with the people who I trusted. Thanks to this firm, the finding of fraud in my case was reversed. I am now a green card holder! Thank you." F.M.

"Quick and efficient but expensive. However, I would never trust any other firm with my case."- J. M.

NEIL RAMBANA

521 East Tennessee Street Tallahassee, Florida 32308

Phone: 866 224 4529

Fax: not available

Website: http://rambanaandricci.com

E-mail: neil@rambana.com

Therapists' Rating		PTSponsor's Rating	
Fees	3	Fees	5
Speed	5	Speed	5
Accessibility	5	Accessibility	5
Overall	4	Overall	5

The Good: The Attorneys at Rambana and Ricci, P.A. are happy to discuss your immigration options with you. However, due to the large number of calls and e-mails we receive, our policy regarding consultations is as follows: The fee for a consultation either in person or via telephone is normally US$150. Consultations last for up to one half hour. The fee must be paid prior to the consultation. It is the potential client's responsibility to contact Rambana & Ricci, P.A. at the appointed time. Our toll-free number is 866 224 4529

The Downside: The fee for a consultation by e-mail is also US$150 which must be paid prior to the consultation and the consultation can include a number of e-mails reasonably calculated to respond to the particular situation of the client. If within one business day of your consultation you decide to hire Rambana and Ricci, P.A. to represent you, the consultation fee will be credited towards the legal fee set for the services we are to provide.

The Bottom Line: There could be both negative and positive reviews for this law firm, chances of getting good service may depend on various circumstances.

Testimonials:"My husband hired this lawyer when he first came to Florida to help get him his green card. BIG MISTAKE! We paid him over $5000 and once he received his payment we were no longer a priority! Did not answer calls, said would send letters but no proof that he did. The firm refused to file a lawsuit for us and Neil refused to speak with us, we had to deal with all the legal flunkies who know less than a rock! I ended up doing the lawsuit myself and got my husband his green card."- N. A.

"I called Rambana & Ricci in a panic a couple of months ago. I had an urgent situation and they were able to answer all of my questions over the phone quickly and professionally. What a relief!! I have been trying for years to acquire my alien status with no avail until I was referred to Rambana & Ricci. What a blessing. They were professional, courteous and extremely knowledgeable. I am proud to say, because of them, I am Florida resident. Thank you"- R. A.

LAW OFFICES OF RV REDDY

Houston, Texas

Phone: 713-953-7787   Fax: not available

Website: www.rvreddy.com   E-mail: emily@rvreddy.com

Therapists' Rating   PTSponsor's Rating

Fees   2   Fees   2

Speed   5   Speed   5

Accessibility 5   Accessibility 5

Overall   4   Overall   4

The Good: They respond immediately. They are also knowledgeable.

The Bad: The legal fee for H1B is more or less $1, 000; on the other hand, the fee for green card is more or less $ 4, 000. The USCIS fee is not included on these quotes.

The Bottom Line: They charge reasonably, plus the speed and accessibility factor.

Testimonial: "This lawyer is affordable!"- R. C.

LAW OFFICES OF SPAR AND BERNSTEIN

225 Broadway, 5th Floor, New York, NY 10007

Phone: 1-800-LAW-LINK   Fax: not available

Website: http://www.4immigration.com   E-mail: info@lawsb.com

Therapists' Rating   PTSponsor's Rating

Fees   2.5   Fees   3

Speed   2.5   Speed   3

Accessibility 2.5   Accessibility 3

Overall   2.5   Overall   3

Testimonials: "I have been very disappointed with the Law Office of Spar & Bernstein. My case is complicated and I received a promise that did not come true. They are very expensive but the price would be worth it if the service was above par. I can never get a paralegal on the phone when I have a question. If I do get one, I won't get the same one twice. The receptionists are not even the slightest bit polite or helpful. I am incredibly disappointed with my whole experience (client since 2003)."- R. Y.

"Mr. Bernstein is the best!! Before I came to see him, I thought I was out of luck. I consulted with him and he didn't just answer all of my questions, he even told me all of the other options available to me which I never thought I was eligible for. After reviewing my case thoroughly, he realized that I should have received my green card years ago have I used my other options which obviously were not known to my prior attorneys. He really knows what he's saying. Now I am a green card holder and I have Mr. Bernstein and his staff to thank for. Thank you so much Mr. Bernstein. I have referred a lot of my friends to you for legal advice and they always come back thanking me for guiding them to the right person."- M. K.

"If you need some straight answers, this is the lawyer to go to. He is very knowledgeable and very honest. He will give you the answer to all your immigration questions, good or bad. I have consulted with other immigration lawyers before I went to see him, and so far he is the most experienced, informed, and up to date with all the immigration issues. My case was complicated to say the least but after I saw him I didn't have to see another attorney - I got all the answers I need and all the help I was looking for." - M. E.

GERMAN T. FLORES

Canterbury Park 246 N. Orem Boulevard Orem, UT 84057

Phone: 801-226-8811

Fax: not available

Website: not available

E-mail: not available

Therapists' Rating

PTSponsor's Rating

Fees 4.5

Fees 5

Speed	1	Speed	1
Accessibility	1	Accessibility	1
Overall	2	Overall	2

The Good: unable to rate accurately

The Downside: This lawyer has been getting a lot of negative reviews from former clients.

The Bottom Line: We attempted to call this lawyer: 1st time: voice mail. The 2nd time: rude receptionist answered, and stated "we don't provide information over the phone."

KENNETH J. ROBINSON

39577 Woodward Ave Ste 300 Bloomfield Hills, MI 48304-5086

Phone: 614-884-4800   Fax: (248) 737-6089

Website: not available   E-mail: not available

RATINGS (therapists' reviews are not yet available for this lawyer)

PTSponsor's Rating

Fees	2
Speed	5
Accessibility	5
Overall	4

The Good: They have offices in Columbus and Springfield. They offer initial telephone consultations for potential new clients. We talked to them and they are very friendly. There is less than 5 minute wait to speak to a lawyer.

The Downside: for H1B legal fees, they charge $ 2,000, while for green card they charge $ 5,000.

The Bottom Line: They seem to be one of the friendliest lawyers we talked to. They are also very informative.

JOANNA M. SCHAFFER

445 Hamilton Avenue, Suite 1102 White Plains, NY 10601 (main office)

Phone: 914-949-7755   Fax: (866) 833-9130

Website: www.visalawusa.com   E-mail: info@visalawusa.com

RATINGS (therapists' reviews are not yet available for this lawyer)

PTSponsor's Rating

Fees   5

Speed   1

Accessibility   1

Overall   2

The Good: (Information from their website): When you engage the firm, you can count on knowledge and experience. Ms. Schaffer has represented clients in a broad range of immigration matters, including nonimmigrant (i.e., temporary) visas, immigrant (i.e., permanent residence, or "green card") visas, citizenship, and deportation /removal proceedings. In addition, she taught immigration law at Baruch College, City University of New York, at the Continuing Studies Division. Ms. Schaffer is a member of the American Immigration Lawyers Association, and currently co-chairs the Immigration Law Committee of the Westchester Women's Bar Association. An immigrant herself, Ms. Schaffer is passionate about making a difference in the lives of her clients. This translates into the highest level of attention to each client's case and understanding each client's needs throughout the complex immigration process. For the convenience of our clients, we maintain two offices: in White Plains, NY (main office), and in midtown Manhattan (Helmsley Building). We understand that time matters, and, in addition to in-person meetings, we offer other convenient ways to work with us: e-mail, phone, fax, and overnight delivery. Finally, our fees are reasonable and based on flat rates, rather than on hourly billing. This allows clients to know the total legal fees in advance. In addition, to further accommodate our clients, we offer payment plans, making our services more affordable.

The Downside: Accurate assessment for the lawyer has not been done.

The Bottom Line: We contacted this law firm and a receptionist answered. They just said point blank that they do not provide quotes over the phone.

LAW OFFICES OF JACOB J. SAPOCHNICK

1552 Sixth Avenue, Suite 5 San Diego, CA 92101

Phone: 619-819-9204   Fax: 619-3930467

Website: www.h1b.biz   E-mail: info@h1b.biz

RATINGS (therapists' reviews are not yet available for this lawyer)

PTSponsor's Rating

Fees   5

Speed   5

Accessibility   5

Overall   5

The Good: The Law Offices of Jacob J. Sapochnik offers straightforward quotes, with immediate response. You don't have to wait for a long time before they respond.

The Downside: They charge $ 3,500 for H1B legal fees. For green card, it is $ 6,000.

The Bottom Line: If you want fast and reliable service, they can be very good, however, they are expensive.

LAW OFFICES OF MOSHE YOUNG AND CRAIG RENETZKY

11900 Ventura Blvd Studio City, CA 91604

Phone: 818-888-5000   Fax: not available

Website: http://www.immigration-attorney-losangeles.com/

E-mail: info@usimmlaw.net

RATINGS (therapists' reviews are not yet available for this lawyer)

PTSponsor's Rating

Fees   5

Speed   5

Accessibility 1

Overall   4

The Good: (Information from their website): The Law Offices of Moshe A. Young consist of 2 attorneys and a full office staff. The attorneys, Moshe A. Young and Craig Renetzky, handle all facets of immigration law including: Citizenship & Naturalization Criminal Related Immigration Deportation & Removal Executive & Professional Work Visas Temporary Visas & Green Cards Mr. Young has appeared in numerous immigration courts throughout California, and in other states. He has handled thousands of immigration matters of all

kinds ranging from appeals, mandamus actions, deportation/removal hearings. These include numerous immigration petitions for green cards, visas, citizenship etc. An immigrant himself, Mr. Young has also seen the process firsthand in his own case, and that of his wife's. Working as the in house Criminal Immigration expert, Craig Renetzky is an experienced criminal defense attorney, having practiced with the Los Angeles County District Attorney's

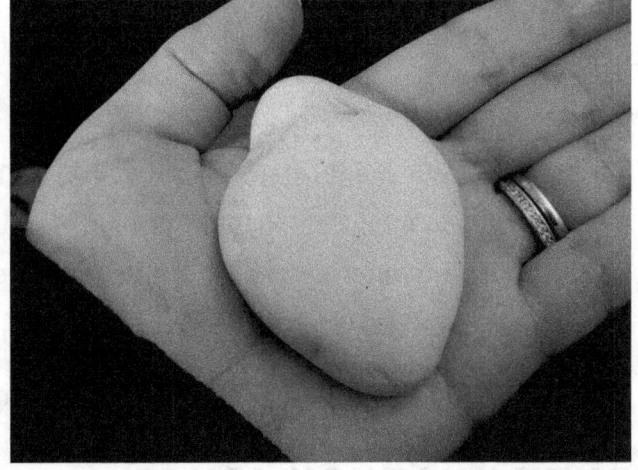

Office for 15 years. Craig Renetzky has handled tens of thousands of criminal cases. He has successfully tried over 100 jury trials, and isn't afraid to defend you all the way to a jury trial and verdict! The Law Offices of Moshe A. Young has a staff that speaks Spanish,

Armenian, Arabic, and Hebrew.

The Downside: We are unable to accurately assess this lawyer.

The Bottom Line: We called this law firm. A receptionist answered the phone. This lawyer was able to call us back the same day, but we were unable to talk to him.

LEIBL & KIRKWOOD

12865 Point Del Mar, Suite 190 Del Mar, CA 92014

Phone: 858-481-5211   Fax: 8584817271

Website: www.usimmigrationlaw.net

E-mail: questions@usimmigrationlaw.net

RATINGS (therapists' reviews are not yet available for this lawyer)

PTSponsor's Rating

Fees	2
Speed	5
Accessibility	5
Overall	4

The Good: Their legal fee for an H1b is $1700. It is cheap, but non-refundable. With the H1B quota, you might be paying the legal fee without any guarantee of getting the H1b. Receptionist answers the phone, but you get a call back within 24 hours.

The Downside: Quotes for a green card depends on your situation.

The Bottom Line: This is an average immigration law firm. They have good response time, and accessibility.

RUTH WALTUCH JONAS

9 Mott Ave # 210 Norwalk, CT 06850-3338

Phone: (203) 852-0333   Fax: (203) 838-1299

Website: not available   E-mail: not available

RATINGS (therapists' reviews are not yet available for this lawyer)

PTSponsor's Rating

Fees   5

Speed   1

Accessibility 1

Overall   2

The Good: unable to provide accurate rating

The Downside: unable to provide accurate rating

The Bottom Line: We contacted this lawyer multiple times, but all we got is the answering machine. (Lawyers, n.d.)

***If you want to be included on our lawyers and agencies list, please send us an email on our website.

About PTSponsor.com

Founded in 2007, PTSponsor was created to provide the most up-to-date information about the Physical Therapy Licensure Process, the National Physical Therapy Exam and the Immigration of Physical Therapists into the U.S. We are dedicated to physical therapists only.

Physical therapists can easily access jobs and information all in one place. Our NPTE section provides the latest tips and reviewers available in the market. Our Immigration section differentiates between tourist visa, H1b (non-immigrant working) visa and immigrant (green card) visa. We constantly update our site for the current visa status, processing dates and case status.

Our resources section has 2 very important parts worth mentioning—best states and expense tracker. The "best states" compares the cost of living, salary and license requirements of each state. The expense tracker provides you an estimate of how much you might spend. The tracker calculates the license fees, FSBPT exam fees, English proficiency exam fees and credentialing fees.

We constantly update our articles to provide you the most recent information on –resume writing, retrogression, CLEP (College Level Examination Program), DMP (Deficiency Make-up Program), Median annual wage (salary) for all the states and much more...

Services

PTSponsor.com now has its very own NPTE Reviewer. If you want to try our exam first, we have included a free practice exam with 25 questions. All you have is to register and you can take the FREE practice test. But in order to access the 30 exams, you have to pay the fee. PTsponsor.com works best with Mozilla Firefox as your web browser. For system requirements, please refer to our website.

PTSponsor allows all registered users to take 30 exams in a month for $30.00 only!

Here is how it works:

1.   Register on our website for a small fee of $30.00.

2.   Once registered you can take the exam.

3.   As long as you are registered, you can take any exam any time. All questions, answers and rationales (if available) can viewed immediately after the exam (not the missed questions only). The new interface will allow you to view all the questions or one question at a time while taking the exam. You are allowed unlimited takes on each exam, until you pass (75%). Your account will expire in 3 months from the time you registered and pay.

Important NPTE Reviewers (National Physical Therapy Exam Reviewers):

1.   International Education Resources- The 2010 NPTE Review & Study Guide , by Susan O'Sullivan and Raymond Siegelman, helps you prepare for the NPTE with a comprehensive review of physical therapy content, study and test-taking strategies, state licensure information, and three complete simulated exams on CD. Rationales and critical reasoning strategies accompany each practice question and help pinpoint your areas of weakness and focus your studying.

Contact details:

500 Davis Street Suite 512 Evanston, IL 60201

Phone: (888)-369-0743   Fax: (847) 328-5049

Web address: www.therapyed.com   Email: info@therapyed.com

Read this book at least 5 times one month before taking the exam.

2.   Score Builders: PTEXAM: The Complete Study Guide

Utilize our comprehensive academic review and then perfect your skills on five full-length sample exams — more questions than any other review product. Our clinically oriented questions prepare you for the rigor of the actual exam and offer an ideal method to determine your current strengths and weaknesses. An extensive academic review and powerful study tools provide candidates with an ideal opportunity to prepare for the breadth and depth of the current examination. An enclosed CD-ROM* allows candidates to experience the various nuances of computer-based testing while assisting them to determine their readiness to take the actual examination.

Contact details:

Phone: (866)-PTEXAMS   Fax: (207) 885-0304

Web address: www.scorebuilders.com   Email: info@scorebuilders.com

This book will get you acquainted with the question and answer format of the exam.

3.   Magee: Orthopedic Physical Assessment by David J. Magee

A systematic approach to performing a neuromusculoskeletal assessment and understanding the reasoning behind various aspects of the assessment. Coverage of every joint of the body, as well as chapters on specific areas such as principles of assessment, head and face, gait, posture, emergency care, and pre-participation evaluation. A CD-ROM that contains an observational gait analysis tool.

This book contains a lot of special tests specific to a particular condition.

4.   Kisner: Therapeutic Exercise: Foundations and Techniques by Carolyn Kisner, Lynn Allen Colby Focuses on all basic therapeutic exercises used for the treatment of musculoskeletal and cardiopulmonary disorders * Covers isokinetics, soft tissue injury repair, surgical procedures, exercise rehabilitation, postoperative management, and posture * Describes functional exercises and exercises that improve functional activities, including closed chain, plyometric, and stabilization exercises * Identifies functional limitations/disabilities as well as structural problems for each diagnosis * Provides guidelines and rationales for choosing and following appropriate exercise procedures. Important exercises are covered in this book.

5.   Sullivan - Physical Rehabilitation: Assessment and Treatment by Susan B. O'Sullivan, Thomas J. Schmitz

Important Topics from our survey:

1. Special Tests, peripheral nerve injuries, upper limb tension test

2. Dermatomal Distribution, spinal cord injuries, cranial nerves, synergies, hemiplegia

3. Glides, Mobilizations, postural drainage

4. Wounds, phases of gait: muscles and foot positions

5. Orthoses and Prostheses: gait deviations associated with improper fitting devices, types of wheelchair for specific diseases or spinal cord injuries

6. Diabetes and insulin; kegel exercises; nephritis and prostate pathology; hypo and hyperthyroidism

7. Fractures: affected nerves, structures and rehabilitation

Other reviewers worth mentioning:
PEAT (On-Line Practice Exam & Assessment Tool)
Federation State Boards of Physical Therapy
509 Wythe Street Alexandria, VA 22314
Phone: (703) 299-3100 Web address: http://www.fsbpt.com
Email: custserv@fsbpt.org

Therapy Team Educational Services, Inc.
823 S. Western Ave Chicago IL 60612
Phone: (877) 476-6684 Fax: (312) 455-0183
Web address: http://www.therapyteam.com Email: therapyteam@hotmail.com

Jane Worley
Director, PTA Program Lake Superior College
2101 Trinity Rd Duluth MN 55811
PTA Basic Refresher Course On-line

Phone: 800-432-2884 ext. 7632

Fax: (218) 733-5937

Web address: http://www.lsc.mnscu.edu

Email: j.worley@lsc.mnscu.edu

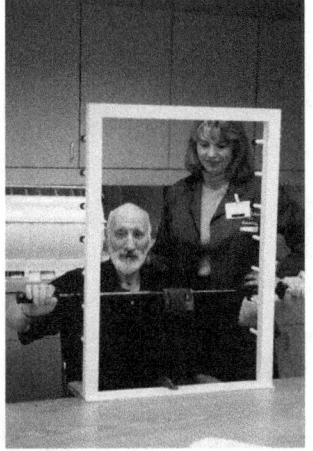

Advanced PT Concepts A+ PT Exam Prep

2495 E. Stephens Road Gilbert, AZ 85296

Phone: (480) 203-5814 Fax: (480) 557-0808

Web address: http://www.apluspt.com Email: info@apluspt.com

PTSponsor.com does not warrant the accuracy or validity of the information and hereby disclaims any liability to any person for any loss or damage caused by errors or omissions in the site. PTSponsor.com also is not responsible for any material or information contained in the linked sites provided. The information presented at this site should not be construed to be formal legal advice or the formation of any relationship.

LIST OF STATES THAT REQUIRE JURISPRUDENCE EXAMS (THROUGH FSBPT)

- Alabama

- Arizona

- California

- District of Columbia

- Florida

- Georgia

- Nebraska

- Ohio

Retrogression and the Schedule A Profession

On November 1, 2006, the Department of State enacted retrogression for Schedule A nurses and physical therapists. Retrogression refers to the resulting delay in obtaining an immigrant visa when there are more people applying for immigrant visas in a given year than the total number of visas available. The applicant cannot file an Application to Adjust Status (Form I-485) or obtain an immigrant visa by attending an immigrant visa interview at a U.S. Consulate abroad. Applicants must wait in line until the immigrant visa becomes available.

For Schedule A petitions, the priority date is the date the Immigrant Petition for Alien Worker (form I-140) was received by the USCIS. Each month, the U.S. Department of State issues a "Visa Bulletin" which announces the priority dates eligible for immigrant visas in each category. This information can be found at the U.S. Department of State website http://travel.state.gov/visa/frvi/bulletin/bulletin_4177.html

Immigrant visa petitions for Schedule A occupations generally fall within the "EB-3" category. This category has been "retrogressed" since 2005. An applicant in this category must have a priority date of April 22, 2001 to July 1, 2005 depending upon their country of birth. However, legislation passed in 2005 allocated an additional 50,000 immigrant visas specifically for Schedule A petitions and created a new EB-3 subcategory, "EX" for these visas. Unfortunately, this special allocation of 50,000 immigrant visas is exhausted. The priority date for the EX category is October 1, 2005. Therefore, as of November 1, 2005, an applicant for an immigrant visa based upon a Schedule A petition would have needed to have filed the I-140 petition on or before October 1, 2005 to be immediately eligible for an immigrant visa.

U.S. Consulates will not assign interview dates and will not be able to issue immigrant visas to Nurses and Physical Therapists until retrogression for Schedule A category ("EX") is resolved. As of November 1, 2005, the ability to "concurrently file" the I-140 and I-485 will be temporarily unavailable. An I-140 petition can still be filed, but the Application to Adjust Status (Form I-485) which provides authorization to remaining the United States and eligibility for employment authorization cannot be filed.

Reference:
United States Citizenship and Immigration Services. www.uscis.gov
"Before contacting the USCIS, USCIS may be able to help you if you have a question about immigration procedures, or need clarification, by calling the USCIS National Customer Service Center (NCSC) at 1-800-375-5283 (TTY 1-800-767-1833). This toll-free call center has additional information and, during their specified office hours, can connect you to live assistance in English and Spanish. The NCSC will be able to answer most questions - although they cannot provide information about the status of your case over the telephone."
PTSponsor.com does not warrant the accuracy or validity of the information and hereby disclaims any liability to any person for any loss or damage caused by errors or omissions in the site. PTSponsor.com also is not responsible for any material or information contained in the linked sites provided. The information presented at this site should not be construed to be formal legal advice or the formation of any relationship.

IMPORTANT CONTACTS PRE-LICENSURE

Immigration

Service	Processing Time	Fees
H1b Visa for PT	15-180 days	$320.00 - $2320.00
H1b Transfer or Renewal	15-180 days	$320.00 - $1870.00
Green Card (I-140) for PT	4-8 months	$475.00
Adjustment of Status (I-485)	1-2 years	$1010.00

Proficiency Exams

Service	Processing Time	Fees
TOEFL	Depends on either PBT/CBT/iBT	$140.00-$200.00
TWE	Included in TOEFL exam	$50.00 for rescore

Credentialing Agencies

Agency	Processing Time	Fees
International Credentialing Associates 7245 Bryan Dairy Road Bryan Dairy Business Park II Largo, FL 33777 Phone: (727)549-8555; (727)549-8555 Fax: (727)549-8554	12 weeks	$425.00
International Consultants of Delaware, Inc P.O. Box 8629 Philadelphia, PA 19101-8629 TEL: (215) 222-8454; (215) 222-8454 ext. 510 FAX: (215) 349-0026 Web site: www.icdel.com E-mail: icd@icdel.com	14 days	$225.00-$500.00

Agency	Processing Time	Fees
Educational Credential Evaluators, Inc. PO Box 514070 Milwaukee WI 53203-3470 USA 414-289-3400; 414-289-3400 eval@ece.org	1, 5, or 12 business days (depending on the type of service you choose)	$325.00-$520.00
FOREIGN CREDENTIALING COMMISSION ON PHYSICAL THERAPY 511 Wythe Street, Alexandria, Virginia 22314-1917 Telephone: 703-684-8406; 703-684-8406 Fax: 703-684-8715	16 weeks	$750.00
International Education Research Foundation, Inc. Post Office Box 3665 Culver City, CA 90231-3665 Phone: 310.258.9451; 310.258.9451 Fax: 310.342.7086	At least 60 days	$350.00

About the TOEFL iBT™ Test. (2010). Educational Testing Services. Retrieved August 10, 2010, from http://www.ets.org/toefl/ibt/about

About the TOEFL® PBT Test. (2010). Educational Testing Services. Retrieved August 10, 2010, from http://www.ets.org/toefl/pbt/about

Agencies. (n.d). PTSponsor-Foreign Trained Physical Therapists' Online Community. Retrieved August 1, 2010, from http://www.ptsponsor.com/all_agencies.php

Alternate identification number, a substitute for a U.S. social security number?. (2008 June 14). PTSponsor. Retrieved August 29, 2010, from http://www.ptsponsor.com/articles.php?page=&catg=#Alternate Identification Number, a Substitute for a U.S. Social Security Number?

Choosing an Agency to Sponsor you for a Visa. (2008 January 26). PTSponsor-Foreign Trained Physical Therapists' Online Community. Retrieved August 1, 2010, from http://www.ptsponsor.com/articles.php?page=&catg=#Choosing an Agency

College Level Examination Program (CLEP). (2008 April 2). PTSponsor-Foreign Trained Physical Therapists' Online Community. Retrieved September 1, 2010, from http://www.ptsponsor.com/articles.php?page=&catg=#College Level Examination Program (CLEP)

Credentials Evaluation Service. (2010 July 16). Commission on Graduates of Foreign Nursing Schools. Retrieved August 1, 2010, from http://cgfns.org/sections/programs/ces/

Credentialing Problems. (2008 April 19). PTSponsor-Foreign Trained Physical Therapists' Online Community. Retrieved September 1, 2010, from http://www.ptsponsor.com/articles.php?page=&catg=#Credentialing Problems

Credential Verification Service for New York State. (2010 July 16). Commission on Graduates of Foreign Nursing Schools. Retrieved August 1, 2010, from http://cgfns.org/sections/programs/cvs/

Evaluation Services. (n.d.). Educational Credentials Evaluators. Retrieved September

8, 2010, from http://www.ece.org/main/content=EvaluationServices&SubSite=1&LeftNav=2

FSBPT Suspends NPTE Examination for All Graduates of Certain Overseas Programs in Response to Pervasive Security Breaches. (2010 August 25). Federation of State Boards on Physical Therapy. Retrieved August 26, 2010 from https://www.fsbpt.org/NewsAndEvents/SecurityBreach20100712/

Fee Schedule. (n.d.). International Consultants of Delaware, Inc. Retrieved September 8, 2010, from http://www.icdeval.com/fees.shtml

Fee schedule and payment information. (2010 July 16). Commission on Graduates of Foreign Nursing Schools. Retrieved August 1, 2010, from http://cgfns.org/sections/apply/fees.shtml

Frequently Asked Questions. (n.d.). Educational Credentials Evaluators. Retrieved September 8, 2010, from http://www.ece.org/main/content=IndividualFAQ&SubSite=1&LeftNav=5

Frequently Asked Questions. (n.d.).Foreign Credentialing Commission on Physical Therapy. Retrieved August 1, 2010, from http://www.fccpt.org/GeneralInformation/FAQs/index.asp

General Information. (n.d.).Foreign Credentialing Commission on Physical Therapy. Retrieved August 1, 2010, from http://www.fccpt.org/GeneralInformation/index.asp

Green Card for Physical Therapists. (). Retrieved September 1, 2010 from http://www.ptsponsor.com/green_card.php

Green Card Through a Job. (2009 December 10). Retrieved August 20, 2010 from http://www.uscis.gov/portal/site/uscis/menuitem.eb1d4c2a3e5b9ac89243c6a 7543f6d1a/?vgnextoid=24b0a6c515083210VgnVCM100000082ca60aRCRD&v gnextchannel=24b0a6c515083210VgnVCM100000082ca60aRCRD

H-1B Visa for Physical Therapists. (2010 May). Retrieved September 1, 2010 from http://www.ptsponsor.com/h1bvisa.php

ICD Physical Therapy and Physical Therapy Assistant Credentials Evaluations for applicants educated outside the United States. (n.d.). International Consultants of Delaware, Inc. Retrieved September 8, 2010, from http://www.icdeval.com/evaluation/physicaleval.shtml

Important Contacts Pre-Licensure. (2008 January 26). PTSponsor-Foreign Trained Physical Therapists' Online Community. Retrieved August 1, 2010, from http://www.ptsponsor.com/articles.php?page=&catg=#Important%20Contacts%20Pre-licensure

Jurisprudence Examinations. (n.d.). Federation of State Boards on Physical Therapy. Retrieved July 20, 2010, from https://www.fsbpt.org/ForCandidatesAndLicensees/Jurisprudence/index.asp

Lawyers. (n.d). PTSponsor-Foreign Trained Physical Therapists' Online Community. Retrieved August 1, 2010, from http://www.ptsponsor.com/all_lawyers.php

NPTE Candidate Handbook . (2010). Retrieved August 10,2010 from https://www.fsbpt.org/ForCandidatesAndLicensees/NPTE/

Overview of the Primary Services. (n.d.).Foreign Credentialing Commission on Physical Therapy. Retrieved August 1, 2010, from http://www.fccpt.org/GeneralInformation/PrimaryServices/index.asp

Overview of the Related Services. (n.d.).Foreign Credentialing Commission on Physical Therapy. Retrieved August 1, 2010, from http://www.fccpt.org/GeneralInformation/RelatedServices/index.asp

Permanent Placement vs. Travelling (2008 July 10). PTSponsor-Foreign Trained Physical Therapists' Online Community. Retrieved July 6, 2010 from http://www.ptsponsor.com/articles.php?page=&catg=#Permanent Placement versus Traveling

Petition for a Nonimmigrant Worker. (2010 September 2). Retrieved September 5, 2010 from http://www.uscis.gov/portal/site/uscis/menuitem.5af9bb95919f35e66f61417543f6d1a/?vgnextoid=f56e4154d7b3d010VgnVCM10000048f3d6a1RCRD&vg nextchanel=7d316c0b4c3bf110VgnVCM1000004718190aRCRD

Physical Therapist. (n.d.). In Wikipedia, The Free Encyclopedia. Retrieved July 13, 2010, from http://en.wikipedia.org/wiki/Physical_therapist

Physical Therapists - The Process (n.d.). Interfysio. Retrieved August 2, 2010, from http://www.interfysio.com/physical-therapists/index.php

Physical Therapy. (2003). The Encyclopedia Americana. Grolier Inc. Danbury: CT. 48-49.

Physical Therapy State Boards Recognizing ICD as a Provider. (n.d.). International Consultants of Delaware, Inc. Retrieved September 8, 2010, from http://www.icdeval.com/who/ptstateboards.shtml

Preparing a Resume. (2008 January 26). PTSponsor-Foreign Trained Physical Therapists' Online Community. Retrieved August 1, 2010, from http://www.ptsponsor.com/articles.php?page=&catg=#Preparing a Resume

Retrogression and the Schedule A Profession. (2008 April 9). PTSponsor-Foreign Trained Physical Therapists' Online Community. Retrieved August 1, 2010, from http://www.ptsponsor.com/articles.php?page=&catg=#Retrogression%20and%20the%20Schedule%20A%20Profession

Social Security number. (n.d.). In Wikipedia-The Free Encyclopedia. Retrieved August 3, 2010, from http://en.wikipedia.org/wiki/Social_Security_number

Social Security Number for Non-Citizens or Foreign Workers. (2008 March 20). PTSponsor-Foreign Trained Physical Therapists' Online Community. Retrieved September 1, 2010, from http://www.ptsponsor.com/articles.php?page=&catg=#Social Security Number for Non-Citizens or Foreign Workers

States. (n.d) PTSponsor-Foreign Trained Physical Therapists' Online Community. Retrieved August 1, 2010, from http://www.ptsponsor.com/all_states.php

Temporary (Nonimmigrant) Workers. (2010 August 10). Retrieved August 20, 2010 from http://www.uscis.gov/portal/site/uscis/menuitem.

Test of Written English Guide. (2004). Educational Testing Service. 5, 4-6, Appendix A.

www.ingramcontent.com/pod-product-compliance
Lightning Source LLC
Chambersburg PA
CBHW081126170526
45165CB00008B/2566